Morning **Pilates** *Workouts*

Cathleen Murakami

Human Kinetics

Library of Congress Cataloging-in-Publication Data

Murakami, Cathleen, 1957-
  Morning Pilates workouts / Cathleen Murakami.
    p. cm.
  Includes bibliographical references and index.
  ISBN-13: 978-0-7360-5954-1 (soft cover)
  ISBN-10: 0-7360-5954-7 (soft cover)
  1. Pilates method. I. Title.
  RA781.4.M87 2007
  613.7'1--dc22

                        2006018821

ISBN-10: 0-7360-5954-7
ISBN-13: 978-0-7360-5954-1

Guidelines from Dr. Cedric Bryant on page 43 reprinted, by permission, from the American Council on Exercise.

The Web addresses cited in this text were current as of June 1, 2006, unless otherwise noted.

Acquisitions Editors: Martin Barnard and Jason Muzinic; **Developmental Editor:** Amanda Eastin; **Assistant Editor:** Christine Horger; **Copyeditor:** Joanna Hatzopoulos; **Proofreader:** Kathy Bennett; **Indexers:** Robert and Cynthia Swanson; **Permission Manager:** Carly Breeding; **Graphic Designer:** Bob Reuther; **Graphic Artist:** Tara Welsch; **Photo Managers:** Dan Wendt and Joe Jovanovich; **Cover Designer:** Keith Blomberg; **Photographer (cover):** © K. Vey/Jump; **Photographer (interior):** Bob Bretell; **Printer:** United Graphics

Human Kinetics books are available at special discounts for bulk purchase. Special editions or book excerpts can also be created to specification. For details, contact the Special Sales Manager at Human Kinetics.

Printed in the United States of America   10 9 8 7 6 5 4 3 2 1

Human Kinetics
Web site: www.HumanKinetics.com

United States: Human Kinetics
P.O. Box 5076
Champaign, IL 61825-5076
800-747-4457
e-mail: humank@hkusa.com

Canada: Human Kinetics
475 Devonshire Road Unit 100
Windsor, ON N8Y 2L5
800-465-7301 (in Canada only)
e-mail: orders@hkcanada.com

Europe: Human Kinetics
107 Bradford Road
Stanningley
Leeds LS28 6AT, United Kingdom
+44 (0) 113 255 5665
e-mail: hk@hkeurope.com

Australia: Human Kinetics
57A Price Avenue
Lower Mitcham, South Australia 5062
08 8372 0999
e-mail: liaw@hkaustralia.com

New Zealand: Human Kinetics
Division of Sports Distributors NZ Ltd.
P.O. Box 300 226 Albany
North Shore City
Auckland
0064 9 448 1207
e-mail: info@humankinetics.co.nz

I dedicate this book to my mom and dad, Robert and Sachiko Murakami.
I love you both.

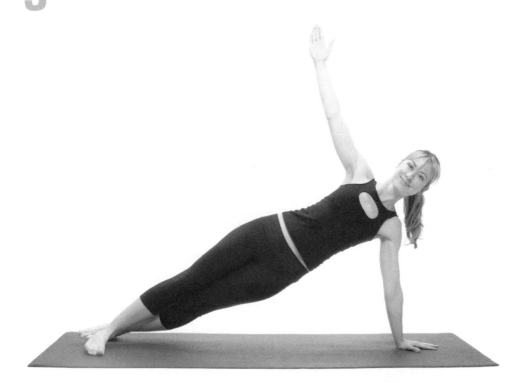

Contents

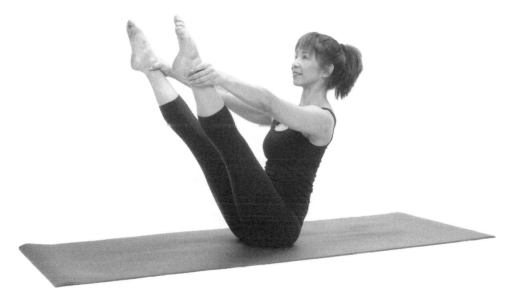

Preface

Congratulations on being a member of the dedicated morning exercise population and on choosing Pilates as your exercise method. Consistent morning exercisers are highly motivated, disciplined, and focused. These attributes serve to keep them on track and feeling fit. As a member of this group, you too share these characteristics. You will reap great rewards from the workouts offered in this book.

Part I contains valuable information designed to give you the most benefit from your morning efforts. Chapter 1 begins with ideas on how to start the day with mental focus and clarity. Ways to keep the mind, body, and spirit optimized through sound sleep habits and intelligent nutritional choices are included along with ways to stay motivated and excited about your workouts. The body feeds the brain and the brain feeds the body, so I share thoughts that will keep that relationship strong and healthy to optimize your workout plan and thus achieve your goals. When you begin to experience the benefits of your consistent morning workout, your motivation level will stay consistent as well.

Having an ideal home workout space, one that meets both your workout needs and creates a mood that will enhance your workout experience, is discussed in chapter 2. I share many options for creatively designing a workout area that is not only functional but also enhances your personal style. Exercising in such an inviting environment will aid you in your dedication and adherence. Your special sanctuary will invite you to enter it even if your space is limited. I am sure you will find yourself looking forward to your daily morning routines and pursuing them with increased conscientiousness, diligence, and enthusiasm. Chapter 2 also covers props, media options, and workout attire.

Chapter 3 provides a discussion of basic anatomy and physiology topics necessary for a functional understanding of the Pilates method. Knowing and understanding these simple yet important aspects of anatomy, body alignment, structure, and muscle function will enrich your exercise efforts and assist you in avoiding injury during workouts and normal daily activities. You already know that Pilates is technique sensitive. The chapter provides some new tidbits of information that will either clarify some key aspects for you or assist you in refining your execution of the exercises themselves. The greater your understanding of your body and how it functions as a whole, the more empowered you will be.

Part II dives right in to the individual exercise routines. Now it's time to get going! In this day and age of cell phones, PDAs, the Internet, and high-speed everything, our lives seem to be getting busier and busier, and time has become a very precious commodity. To help you conduct all the necessary obligations of your daily life and still manage to include some quality exercise time for yourself, the routines are divided into three levels of challenge as well as three time lengths. You can choose from 20-, 40-, and 60-minute routines at either a light-, moderate-, or high-intensity level. So, as your schedule fluctuates, *you* can adapt your workout based on time, energy level, or both. If you have more time, you can choose the 60-minute routine; if you have less time for exercise on one day, you can choose a 20-minute routine. The time frame allowed does not include your optional 5- to 10-minute motor revver (warm-up), so you will need to plan accordingly. At the end of each chapter, the exercises are listed in alphabetical order by name for quick reference. You can find each exercise either by page number or its alphabetical listing.

The routines include classic Pilates exercises such as the hundred, teaser, and swimming. Also included are some perhaps less familiar choices such as control balance, mermaid, and jackknife. You will find yourself moving through some yoga type stretches and transitions as well as challenging yourself with some calisthenic type exercises such as simple push-ups. While your physical strength, flexibility, coordination, and balance improve, you will definitely find your mental strength and flexibility increasing as well.

Joseph Pilates was a pioneer in his thinking about physical and mental fitness. His original 34 mat exercises are the foundation on which the routines in this book are built. I have used most of his user-friendly classics and designed a format that is intelligent and safe in sequence and that smoothly flows from one exercise to the next. You can increase the benefits of many of the exercises simply through stretching a muscle group that might *limit* your range or capability to properly perform it. By incorporating a few simple stretches through smooth transitions, you will not only get more physical benefits, but you will also increase your mental acuity and endurance. Feel free to hold the stretches for longer or add in your own if your schedule allows. The routines in this book are based on my decades of experience in instructing exercise classes. My weekly mat class students serve as guinea pigs for my inventive and imaginative mind, too! As you become accustomed to the exercise regimens I've arranged, you can mix and match routines to customize your workout.

Pilates exercise helps you strengthen the distinct and unbreakable bond between the body and mind. I applaud you for your efforts in getting to this point. I know you will enjoy these routines, and you might even find yourself creatively inspired to mix and match as you fancy. Go for it and enjoy!

Acknowledgments

So many individuals have contributed to my ability to even attempt this project. If I have left anyone out, please forgive my oversight. The following people directly or indirectly contributed to the creation of this book:

My parents have done so much for me. When I was 6 years old, Mom took me to see a ballet in which Rudolf Nureyev and Margot Fonteyn were the principal dancers. It was then that I decided I wanted to become a ballerina, so I begged her for ballet lessons. Thanks to Mom for saying yes, and thanks to Dad for paying for those lessons. Although ballet never paid the rent, it led me to the career of teaching exercise, and I've never looked back.

Joseph Pilates pioneered and manifested his ideas of health and exercise. He was truly ahead of his time.

Martin Barnard of Human Kinetics conceptualized the original book series and believed in me.

Mandy Eastin, my developmental editor at Human Kinetics, contributed her patience, kindness, and support. She reined in my thoughts and offered incredibly perceptive insight and guidance. She encouraged me and acted as my cheering squad when I thought I was drowning. She even allowed me (she had no choice!) to leave long messages on her voice mail in the middle of the night. (Aren't you glad you are on CST, Mandy?)

Bobby Bretell patiently and meticulously took the great photographs that appear throughout the book. Kari Topzand generously provided us with workout outfits that were not only functional but beautifully crafted as well. Jennifer Martin has been my loyal senior trainer at SynergySystems® Fitness Studio, a beautiful model, and my friend. Much love to you, Jenn—we've been through a lot over the years. Yancey Scoggin was a superb model for the shoot, and he "cleaned up" so well! Coco Bennett has been my enthusiastic "sistah," beautiful model, and friend. Amy Goldberg kept my office under control, listened when no one else knew how, and has been my little sister and dear friend when I thought I would implode under the pressures of deadlines and running the business.

Alan Herdman, director of Alan Herdman Studios in London, England, generously trained me as an apprentice out of the goodness of his heart, even though I wore thong leotards in his proper British studio. His brilliant work inspires me still. If it weren't for Alan, I would not be teaching Pilates today. Marie-José Blom-Lawrence, director of Long Beach Dance Conditioning, is my mentor and friend; she trusts me to teach her work and continually inspires me with her genius, humor, and brilliance. Thanks, MJ. You never cease to amaze me. Phyllis Pilgrim believed in me when I first came back from London with so much enthusiasm and nowhere to channel it. Thank you for giving me the opportunity to take the seed that was there and cultivate it into fruition. Deborah Szekeley trusted Phyllis and allowed my dream of a fully equipped Pilates studio to be created at Rancho La

Puerta. Rancho La Puerta provided me with a place where my teaching skills could sharpen, grow, and deepen. It was at the Ranch that I learned to take a complex modality such as Pilates and simplify it for the nonexerciser. Laura Gallerstein, who originally introduced me to Alan, pioneered the Pilates at Rancho La Puerta and did Runes with me that day on the mountain when we knew my life would never be the same again.

IDEA Health & Fitness Association trusted me with the first Pilates presentation at their World Fitness Convention in 1994 (when the mainstream had never heard of Pilates) and has kept me on their presenter roster ever since. Ralph LaForge Exercise Physiologist, Duke University Medical Center, shared his enthusiasm for my teaching with Patti McCord and IDEA. Patti McCord (former educational director for IDEA) believed Ralph when he told her about Pilates and my teaching.

Madeline Black, director of Studio M in Sonoma, California, has been a constant support as a peer and great friend. She is a brilliant teacher in her own right.

Balanced Body has supported me in so many ways since my Ranch days and provided me with the best equipment available on the market today. Chris Kidd provided me with a place to stay during my apprenticeship with Alan. Gillian Cornish allowed me to sleep on her floor in a tiny flat in Willesden Green during my apprenticeship and was my friend during the days when I "didn't get it." She, along with Trevor Blount and Nick Ringham taught me at Alan's.

Thanks from the bottom of my heart to all my past and present students and clients. You have taught me more about myself than I could ever learn on my own.

Most of all I thank the Great Creator for giving me the gift of teaching something I love and believe in so that I might share the little bit I know with the world.

part one

AM Readiness

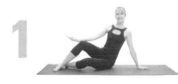

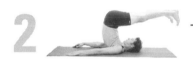

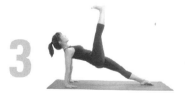

1

Energy to Start the Day

Good morning! As a regular morning exerciser, chances are you just wake up and get up. No hitting the snooze button 14 times, no peering at the clock with one eye barely open, and no groaning for you. When you wake up, you leap out of bed ready to start your day. Okay, perhaps it's not that way for you every single day, but on the whole you probably do like getting up early and getting going before most of the rest of the world does.

After a good night's sleep you most likely have had a mild fast—no intake of food or drink for about 8 to 10 hours. You get a good 6 or 8 hours of sleep in, and much of it is started before midnight. The average person is usually in bed by about 11 p.m., while the dedicated morning exerciser is usually between the sheets at least an hour earlier. Mornings are the time when you feel less cluttered by your day. Your body may be a little bit stiffer but your mind is freer from thoughts, worries, and daily obligations and distractions. With that extra mental energy you are able to concentrate much more fully and with more power than you can later in the day. There just might be something to that old saying, The early bird catches the worm.

This chapter teaches you how to take advantage of your dedication to your regular morning exercise regimen. You are pretty self-motivated and disciplined in the morning; otherwise, you would not have picked up this book. However, some days you might wake up with a little or a lot less motivation than usual despite knowing how much better you feel when you actually get your buns in gear. At times sleep, hydration, nutritional, and mental stumbling blocks can contribute to lethargy, so this chapter provides you with some guidelines that have helped me overcome those challenges. If the guidelines work on the days when you are dragging, just think how charged you will feel on the days when you wake up already strongly motivated!

Rise and Shine!

The early bird may catch the worm, but how does it know when to wake up? The answer is, It operates on circadian rhythm. You may have noticed that birds tend to wake up with the sun and go to sleep at dusk. Plants tend to open their flower petals or leaves during daylight and close again at dusk. Humans operate on circadian rhythms as well. Blood pressure, heart rate, and body temperature all increase upon waking and decrease when sleeping. This rhythm is the routine to which the human body is naturally set. The body is naturally preparing itself to get going. We now live in a society that has the modern-day convenience of electricity and lights, but in the pioneer days of our culture, the day's activities began at the crack of dawn and wound down at sunset. It makes sense that we try to follow the laws of Mother Nature and work with this circadian rhythm. The human body seems to function best with a regular routine for eating, sleeping, and activity. Waking up at the same time every day to get your workout in helps your body to regulate many functions for optimal performance all day long.

Be sure you get adequate rest to rejuvenate yourself for whatever your morning workout might bring your way. Inadequate sleep will leave you less alert and more tired during your workout and as the day progresses. Research has also shown that your body is better able to prepare for the day ahead when your sleeping routine is consistent. In fact, there is increasing evidence that inadequate sleep may in fact be a large contributor to an unhealthy lifestyle.

While we know that Pilates is not a specific weight-loss regimen, the following information might prove relevant in relation to your nutritional habits, especially if you are lacking on the shut-eye. Something you may not have known is that too little sleep may mean too many pounds. Not getting enough sleep can increase blood levels of ghrelin, an appetite-stimulating hormone. Ghrelin, in turn, triggers a *decrease* in the levels of the hormone leptin, which is believed to help control appetite. The result: increased cravings for high-calorie, high-carbohydrate foods. This theory has been confirmed by the following two studies. In the first study (Spiegel et al. 2004), 12 young men were allowed just 4 hours of sleep, 2 nights in a row. Blood measurements showed that the subjects' ghrelin levels rose by 28 percent while leptin levels fell by 19 percent. When the men received adequate sleep, blood levels returned to normal. In a separate study (Taheri et al. 2004), the sleeping patterns and hormone levels of more than 1,000 people were analyzed.

People allowed to sleep fewer than 5 hours a night had 15 percent more ghrelin and 15 percent less leptin than people allowed to sleep at least 8 hours a night.

How might this information apply to you, the dedicated morning Pilates enthusiast? Sleep deprivation, especially on the days when you are exceptionally pressed for time and need to get many things done, could upset the ghrelin and leptin levels in your body and cause you to inadvertently crave high-calorie foods that are empty nutritionally. While the habit of waking up early using your internal clock is a good one, if you went to bed late and did not get enough sleep, you might find yourself also craving sugar to stay awake later in the day. High-carbohydrate foods are not the best choices, especially for the sustained energy you need for a workout as well as for recovery. You can see how essential good sleep is to having sufficient energy for your Pilates workouts and to help you make the best nutritional choices in the morning.

Before you begin your workout, check your mental state. Now is the time to scan your awareness so that the time you spend exercising is optimized and efficient. Are you full of energy? If yes, great! Are you tired? Physical fatigue could be noted as lethargy, heaviness in the limbs, excessive soreness in the muscles or joints, and shakiness. Mental or emotional fatigue could be evidenced with lack of ability to focus or concentrate, irritability, or feeling especially emotionally reactive. If you do not get a good night's sleep that leaves you refreshed upon awakening and are feeling the effects, you may wish to choose either a slightly shorter or less challenging workout for that particular day. For example, if you normally do the 40-minute moderate workout in this book, try doing the 20-minute moderate or light workout.

Suppose you've had less than optimal night's worth of rest and find yourself dragging and craving either caffeine or sugar to keep going. Or, perhaps you are not sleep-deprived but tried a higher-intensity workout and find yourself a bit more fatigued because of the new demand you placed on your body. What can you do to assist yourself in recovery? A nap at some point in the day might be just the perfect choice for you, and it will help you get back in your sleep rhythm the next day. In some studies, a 30-minute nap has been shown to decrease fatigue and increase alertness. Benefits of sneaking in a snooze include the following:

- You can catch up on lack of sleep, whether chronic or a one-time thing.
- It helps to keep those hormones in check, thus maintaining control over your nutritional choices.
- It gives your body some added time for exercise recovery.
- It helps you avoid unnecessary cravings for sugar or caffeine in order to keep functioning.

Europeans and Latin Americans have been taking short daily naps for centuries. For many reasons, the lifestyle in North America doesn't support this practice. For the sleep-deprived person, however, napping or resting during the day for as little as 10 minutes can help. Sometimes you don't even have to be fully sleeping; just lying down with your eyes closed and relaxing the body can do the trick. Find a quiet place where you can fully recline with your body, head, and neck fully supported. If you are on the floor, rest your arms out to the sides as in the yoga pose savasana (also called corpse pose). If you are on a couch or bed, rest your arms on your belly. If you feel pressure in your lower back, bend your knees slightly and place a pillow or support under your knees so that they can rest fully on the support. If you are at work and are unable to get fully supine, consider either putting your feet up on your desk and leaning back in your chair with your eyes closed for a few minutes or going for the kindergarten position of head down on your forearms on top of your desk.

Breathe slowly, and allow yourself to become fully immersed in your rest position. Avoid napping much longer than 45 minutes, because you could awaken feeling more groggy than refreshed. The artist Salvador Dalí held a silver spoon in his hand above a silver tray on his lap. When the spoon fell from his hand and clattered atop the tray, that was all the sleep he needed to feel refreshed! While you may not opt for the silver spoon alarm system, using some sort of an alarm allows you to fully immerse yourself in your rest state because you know that if you happen to completely conk out, your alarm will rouse you.

Water for Your Tank

Nearly two thirds of the human body is water. Water is an essential nutrient that is involved in every function of the body. It helps transport nutrients in and waste products out of cells. It is necessary for all digestive, absorption, circulatory, and excretory functions as well as for assimilating water-soluble vitamins. Water also helps maintain proper body temperature.

Always drink plenty of water. You can live without food for several weeks, but you can go less than a week without water. Water must be continuously replaced in the body. On average, you lose 250 milliliters of water daily just through breathing. The old rule of thumb, eight glasses (or 2 liters) of water a day, is a good minimum. While experts have not agreed on one universal amount, it is accepted that performance declines with dehydration. By drinking an adequate amount of water each day, you can ensure that your body has all it needs to maintain good health. The best way to get water into your body is by drinking plain water. Other beverages, such as fruit juices, milk, and noncaffeinated drinks, can hydrate the body because they contain a high percentage of water. In addition, fruits and vegetables can be good water sources. If you work out in high altitude or a desert environment, both of which will have very low humidity, or if you work out on an exceptionally hot day, remember to boost your minimum intake of clear fluids.

Starting out hydrated is a good choice for morning exercisers. Drink water before your workout; you lose water while you exercise even without heavy perspiration. Ingesting at least a glass of pure water shortly after rising is a good way to hydrate your system. Adding a small squeeze of lemon for taste also helps stimulate the bowels to evacuate soon thereafter, which will help you feel more comfortable during your workout routine.

Many of you are probably morning coffee or tea drinkers. If you must have some caffeine in the morning, go for it—but consider having a large glass of water first. Although many physicians consider caffeine a diuretic, some recent studies have questioned this belief. As with any fluid, coffee may send you to the bathroom a little more frequently, but a major report by the U.S. government's Institute of Medicine concludes that coffee quenches thirst as effectively as water and *does not* deplete bodily fluids (McAuliffe 2005). And, because coffee reduces muscle fatigue and boosts speed and endurance, enjoying a cup of Joe before your workout may enhance your efforts. Sport psychologists attribute these benefits to caffeine's potent ability to release adrenaline, which in turn strengthens muscle contractions and fosters the creation of energy from fatty acids. So, enjoy your cup of coffee or tea in the morning, and get your a.m. boost. It seems to have no negative effect on your hydration, and you can always have a glass of water first just to be sure.

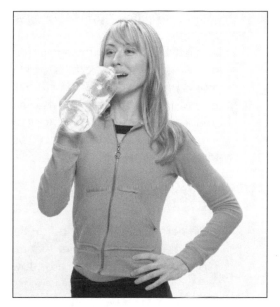

Water is an essential nutrient that is involved in every function of the body. Be sure to hydrate before and after your workout.

Hydration is particularly important for the morning workout enthusiast. Remember, you've just awakened from a 8- to 10-hour fast. Because proper hydration improves the quality of your workout, reduces fatigue, reduces recovery time, and increases your level of satisfaction, it is especially important for you to hydrate yourself before as well as after your workout session. Keep in mind that thirst is not the best scale by which to measure whether or not you are well hydrated. If your urine is the color of lemonade, you're doing well; if by chance it is leaning toward the color of apple juice, you need to reach for another glass of fluid. Also, some symptoms of dehydration are headache, poor concentration, tiredness, and constipation. If you happen to feel you need extra electrolytes because you were sweating excessively, you can mix your own electrolyte cocktail using 1 cup (237 milliliters) plain water, 1 cup orange juice, and a pinch of salt. I personally like those Emergen-C packets by Alacer Corporation. They come in a variety of flavors; they are full of electrolytes, B vitamins, and vitamin C; they taste good; and they are easily portable.

Fuel for the Engine

Discussing morning eating strategies can be tricky. Each body is different, so no one strategy works for everyone. The word "diet" seems to carry a feeling of deprivation for many people. Age, activity level, and stress can greatly affect each person's nutritional needs.

In this section I provide suggestions on what and how much to eat before a morning workout, and I present current information on nutrient timing. Tuning in to what works best for you is part of your journey to self-discovery and empowerment. Use these suggestions to experiment with different approaches and see what works best for you. You may find that what works best for you changes according to the seasons or weather, your age, your environment, and mental stresses that might be occurring in your life. It also depends on what choices you make for your level of workout participation. You might want to consult a qualified nutritionist to explore what eating strategies are right for you.

To Eat or Not to Eat?

Whether you should or shouldn't eat at all before working out is debatable and up to each person. Remember that after you've been sleeping for 6 to 8 hours, your blood sugar level will be a bit low. I have to eat a tiny bit of something before I work out, especially if it's going to be a longer (e.g., 60-minute) session. I usually have half a banana or other type of fruit, a half a cup (118 milliliters) of yogurt, a hard-boiled egg, or a few ounces of a smoothie that I can finish after the workout (my current favorite). I also happen to have an extremely fast metabolism, iron stomach, and blood sugar levels that need to be kept a bit higher. I have learned to consider my physical and mental state and my environment when making a workout choice. With awareness (and sometimes professional guidance), you will, too.

If you exercise soon after you wake up, you probably don't want a large heavy meal in your stomach. Not only does it feel uncomfortable and cause potential gas, but it also makes you feel sluggish and somewhat unmotivated. Eating a large meal causes blood to be shunted to your digestive tract. The very same blood you will need to feed your brain and body during your workout will be busy trying to help digest your food. However, if it happens to be a day when you are not working out immediately, perhaps you wish or need to have a breakfast of a bit more substance because you have the time to allow for it to digest properly before embarking on your workout routine.

For those of you who don't wish or need to have a lot of fuel before working out, or if you are embarking on one of the 20-minute routines, I suggest you hydrate with water upon awakening, opt for your caffeinated or noncaffeinated beverage, and also ingest something similar to the following: a small bit of fruit with yogurt, fruit with egg, a small serving of oatmeal with a dollop of yogurt, or a half a piece of toast with almond butter. I am a big fan of always ingesting a small amount of protein along with whatever else I am having. It levels out my blood sugar and keeps my energy constant.

If those suggestions seem too filling for you or you just don't feel hungry, consider a smoothie. I make one nearly every day when I am working. Smoothies are fast and easy to prepare, and you can always make something different because of the many combinations available to you. Just be creative or choose fruits that are seasonal. Many recipes are available in books and online; just do a search for smoothie recipes. Here is a basic recipe that you can vary by the kind of fruit or liquid base you choose to use. Put the following in a blender or food processor, and blend until smooth:

- 8 to 12 ounces (237 to 355 milliliters) diluted unsweetened cran-water*, pomegranate juice, orange juice, or soy milk
- 1/2 banana
- 1/4 cup (59 milliliters) of fruit (any kind of berry, peaches, mango, or pineapple), fresh or frozen
- 1 or 2 scoops whey protein (I prefer Jay Robb Whey Protein in vanilla flavor, the only one on the market sweetened with stevia, which keeps your system alkaline and does not affect blood sugar), or any other protein powder
- 1 spoonful of yogurt (optional)
- 1 tablespoon flax oil (optional)

*Cran-water is made by diluting 4 ounces (118 milliliters) of unsweetened pure cranberry juice in 32 ounces (almost a pint or liter) of water. I also like to dilute my juices such as pomegranate or orange as well to keep sugar levels down.

Drink a few ounces of your smoothie about 15 minutes before your workout, and finish the rest afterward. The 15 minutes should give you enough time to assimilate what is in your stomach. Some of you will be fine with this amount whether you are just participating in a 20-minute routine or a longer cardio plus 60-minute high-intensity routine. Some of you will prefer or need to ingest a bit more fuel for the longer routines. The following are combinations that you may mix to fuel up for a longer haul:

- 3 to 4 ounces (89 to 118 milliliters) fruit
- 1/2 to 1 cup (118 to 237 milliliters) yogurt with or without granola or mixed into some oatmeal
- Eggs (hard boiled, poached, or scrambled with a variety of vegetables or low-fat cheese and a meat or soy product)
- Ezekiel brand bread toast with almond or peanut butter
- High-protein, low-sugar cold cereal, oatmeal, or granola with fruit

I highly recommend Ann Louise Gittleman's books *The Fat Flush Plan* and *The Fat Flush Cookbook* for additional recipes and ideas. She has many delicious ideas for breakfast and other quick meals that are higher in protein and lower in simple carbohydrate to keep blood sugar levels even, which helps keep your energy on an even keel as well. An added bonus is that your complexion, hair, and nails will also benefit.

Timing Is Everything

There is a recent buzz about nutrient timing and its ability to enhance performance, promote recovery, and improve muscle integrity. The premise behind nutrient timing is to ingest ideal nutrient combinations at optimal times. In other words, realizing the emphasis on *when* to eat as opposed to *what* to eat. The purpose of nutrient timing is to support optimal performance during a training session, provide all that is needed for muscle growth, exploit glycogen replenishment after activity (glycogen is the desired fuel to burn during exercise), and follow a diet that promotes growth and repair around the clock. It is based on data supporting variances in hormonal release throughout the day and in response to exercise. Although nutrient timing appears best suited for competitive athletes, its fundamental strategies can benefit the nonprofessional workout warrior as well. The important and vital relationship between proper nutrition and performance and recovery is something that all professional athletes are aware of. For you, the dedicated independent exerciser, this information might prove its worth in gaining the most from your disciplined morning efforts.

The basic process of nutrient timing is this: Within the 3-hour postworkout time frame, you consume four small meals: an initial liquid meal and three food meals. These meals ideally contain about 40 grams of protein and 20 to 30 grams of carbohydrate each. This combination allows a steady stream of amino acids to be channeled directly toward the goal of feeding your muscles, keeping your body mass lean and providing you with recovery.

Professional athletes who use the anabolic nutrient timing factor (ANTF) approach have full, hydrated, nutrient-dense, and glycogen-filled (energy-filled) muscles. The science behind increasing muscle tissue lies in a complex interaction involving the muscles, liver, and blood. Additionally, the amount of amino acids present in these tissues is a significant factor. This is called anabolism, or an anabolic state—a favorable state in the body created by a combination of good training, nutrition, and rest that leads to increased lean muscle and fat loss, something that all exercisers are interested in maintaining as much as possible. The core of ANTF is nutrient manipulation and stimulation of the pancreas to secrete insulin at the proper time. If you can use this technique, you will be able to keep your body in the muscle-enhancing, fat-reducing, energy-efficient anabolic state. Managing the amount of insulin present in the blood is the key to success in the ANTF approach.

Here are the steps of nutrient timing and the principles behind those steps:

1. *After you finish your workout, elevate your blood sugar levels with a liquid that contains both carbohydrate and protein so that insulin levels increase.* If your blood insulin level is high, the insulin will push the protein into the muscle cells. Insulin has the ability to drive protein and carbohydrate into muscle tissue, but the consumption of protein alone will not stimulate insulin secretion. You need carbohydrate to quickly elevate the blood insulin. The best type of carbohydrate for this purpose should come in liquid form. When trying to elevate blood insulin levels, using a juice containing a high sucrose to fructose ratio is preferable. Grape, orange, or tangerine juices are a few examples of liquid carbohydrate. They provide the bloodstream with a quick surge of amino acids, which is needed immediately after training.

Consuming the prescribed type of carbohydrate at the appropriate time mixed with protein (smoothie, anyone?) creates the optimal anabolic environment. Just as eating protein does not guarantee that the amino acids (building blocks of muscle tissue) will be used to repair muscle tissue, consuming carbohydrate does not guarantee that it will replenish glycogen and provide energy either. So, drinking your smoothie (first postworkout meal, which should have the necessary balance of carbohydrate) will get your insulin secreted to utilize the carbohydrate and thus support the anabolic state to absorb the protein. It's a domino effect: Producing an increase in insulin results in a maximal uptake of glucose and protein. The glucose is transported into the muscle cells and locked inside the muscle as glycogen, which is readily available to energize your next workout.

2. *Within 30 minutes of that liquid ingestion, eat a small low-fat meal that has some protein and carbohydrate.* To keep your energy optimized, consume a second postworkout meal about 30 minutes after ingesting the initial liquid mixture of carbohydrate and protein (that smoothie!). The meal should be low in fat so that it will digest quickly, and it should contain easily absorbed carbohydrate along with a lean source of protein.

The second meal is similar to the first meal in nutrient composition; however, it needs to be in the form of solid food. At this time the best carbohydrate choices would be a baked potato; steamed white rice; cooked grits; or pasta with grilled chicken, fish, or a meat sauce. Eggs are another great choice (especially because it might be what your morning taste buds are seeking), and you can cook them in numerous ways with one of the types of carbohydrate just mentioned as well. Consuming this combination ensures that the amino acids from the protein (whey) in the first meal will be used for continuing the anabolic state and not just the restoration of blood glucose.

3. *In about an hour, have another small meal similar to the second or, if it's too filling, have another small smoothie combo or protein bar.* You're almost there! After consuming the second meal, wait about an hour before ingesting the third. Eating two more small solid food meals similar to the second will optimize what you've already consumed. If you feel too full to eat another meal, opt for another small smoothie with perhaps a half of a potato. Be creative by using any of the other designated types of carbohydrate, but remember that the third meal should be small in content.

4. *Before the 3-hour anabolic window closes, have one last small meal.* Now you have about another 90 minutes to ingest your fourth and final anabolic meal. You could even opt for one of the popular protein bars that are on the market, but I caution you to read the label carefully because many of them are high in simple sugars (e.g., corn syrup). Use your best judgment in deciding when to consume the final meal. Try to ingest it within the last half hour of the anabolic window.

With a few trial runs, you will be able to discern how much and of which foods to choose from and combine.

I know this approach can initially seem daunting. However, if you're a dedicated morning exerciser who is interested in gleaning as much as possible from your disciplined efforts and feeling energized from them, this fully documented method just might give you the added edge on those days when excessive fatigue might affect your attitude and therefore your motivation levels.

Maintaining Motivation

How do you stay motivated, disciplined, or excited about doing a workout that could become boring and repetitive? What about those days when you just feel blah, tired, or too busy? How do you deal when visitors sidetrack you or your job requires extra time and energy for a project? Maybe you feel as though you haven't been achieving the results you had hoped for, or perhaps you are returning from childbirth with the demands of a newborn baby, or a longer-than-usual bout with the flu has you feeling a little bit less than thrilled.

Staying motivated is a lot about your attitude. Having a healthy, positive mindset will enable you to not only get more but also enjoy more out of life. This section presents some of the reasons you might find yourself lacking in motivation and gives you solutions to get you up and moving on the mat. While it's very helpful to know and understand why you might wake up in the doldrums, it's even better to know what choices you have to spring yourself out of them.

Stress

Everyone has worries and responsibilities. Everyone gets overwhelmed by work and family obligations. Financial burdens, children, divorce, career moves, and residential changes are all a part of our fast-paced lives, and these things also can occur simultaneously.

According to Hans Selye, MD, who pioneered the concept of emotional stress, the sympathetic nervous system sets in motion a series of physiological responses to a situation perceived as stressful (1980). Hormones that are produced by the adrenal cortex, including cortisol and epinephrine, prepare the body for an instant state of readiness, more commonly known as the fight-or-flight response. Selye also theorized that once the stress-invoking threat had passed, the body returned to a normal state of balance, called homeostasis. However, recent research shows that when the body chronically pours out stress hormones, it could result in undesirable weight gain. Some researchers believe that chronically elevated cortisol levels can lead to weight gain, especially in the belly area.

This potential weight gain, particularly in the midsection of the body, can hinder your ability to flex the torso forward as well as rotate and twist. The extra "you" just gets in the way! This result is not to be desired, so the sooner you can get a handle on your stress levels, thus managing your hormones, the better. Not only will you feel more agile and adept at your movements, but your body will not feel as heavy and lethargic when exercising.

You can take many safe steps if you are struggling with sticking to your regular morning routine because of life's circumstances (commonly known as stress). While finding a qualified health care practitioner for nutritional guidance and support for dealing with stress and psychotherapy support for some added emotional stresses can be extremely helpful, checking your own ratings on a stress scale could provoke some thought, awareness, and introspection on the role that stress may be playing in your life. You can find a stress scale online by searching for the phrase "life event stress scale."

Exercise improves mood by producing positive biochemical changes in the body and brain. Regular exercise reduces the amount of adrenal hormones your body releases in response to stress. Additionally, with exercise your body releases greater amounts of endorphins, the powerful, pain-relieving, mood-elevating chemicals in the brain. Depressed people often lack these neurochemicals. So, if you've skipped your workout because you are feeling overly stressed, you actually lose out on this very powerful way to alleviate your tension levels.

The mind–body disciplines of exercise are always highly recommended ways to relieve stress because of their effectiveness in clearing or refocusing the mind, which is the first component of adhering to a routine. Because exercise in itself is a great stress reducer, during those occasional moments when anxiety or worries might distract you from your regular adherence to your workout schedule, consider incorporating some of the following suggestions:

- **Work out with a buddy.** Finding a workout partner or group can be extremely helpful. When you have someone with whom you have set workout dates, that partner can often be the factor to get you off your tush and onto your mat. You can probably do the same for your partner at some point as well. The buddy system works wonders when you know another person is waiting for you to get on the mat and you don't want to let the person down. In addition to being helpful when lack of motivation might be sidetracking you, having a regular workout buddy could in fact inspire you to create and attain new fitness goals for yourself.

When you know you are accountable for showing up because of someone else, you are less likely to flake out. The concept of the workout buddy motivates you in a similar way as prepaying for classes. No one likes to lose money when they don't show up for their prepaid class. Just knowing that you have committed to someone who is waiting for you can sometimes be that extra boost you need to actually get out of bed and *move*. Sometimes with all the changes that life throws your way, having the one consistent factor of a buddy to exercise with can be the lifesaver in a whirlwind of events.

If your workout buddy joins you for your initial cardio warm-up, chatting together and sharing some of the load just might help to alleviate some of the burden you have been experiencing. I have found that a sympathetic ear seems to lighten and brighten my outlook, and the outside perspective can sometimes help me to stop sweating the small stuff.

• **Add some cardio.** Because you have been a dedicated morning exerciser, you already are well aware of the benefits of "just doing it." You've probably heard of how the body secretes endorphins, which give you an overall sense of well-being and peace; in other words, they help you feel less stressed. This effect (sometimes referred to as "runner's high") also occurs when you engage in mild to vigorous cardiovascular activity as well as meditation. So, perhaps adding in one or both of these activities either before or after your chosen morning Pilates routine might help you deal with extra stress in your life.

Consider adding in a little cardio (a light walk if you have low energy; a light run if you have higher energy) before your Pilates routine and then a 5- to 10-minute meditation at the end. Or, perhaps do a little cardio or meditation later on in your day if your schedule allows for it. Even if you don't add it in at the same time, you still get the benefits. In fact, because the endorphin secretion is spread out (you do get some endorphin release from your Pilates routine), your state of well-being lasts longer, thus helping you keep a positive attitude between workouts.

• **Meditate.** I know from experience that setting aside quiet time for myself each day, even if it is just a few minutes, helps me stay grounded, centered, and less tightly wound. Exercise has been shown to improve the mental state, from a general mood lift to lessening the symptoms of severe depression. A positive mental state is ideal for meditation, and meditation can make the most of a positive mental state. Mind–body fitness is the ultimate fitness goal, and it is the only true complete approach. I think meditation should be as integral to your fitness program as other components of your workout routine. Your mind is a powerful ally in healing as well as in focusing, and meditation keeps the mind primed. Just like the body, the mind needs to stay flexible and strong.

Bear in mind that if you are already feeling overwhelmed, *adding* to your current schedule could potentially throw you off even more—especially if you have a more driven, type A personality to begin with. I suggest that you incorporate some of the stress-relief techniques if you can be comfortable figuring out how to include them into your morning equation. If you find that adding in the cardio or meditation seems to create *more* anxiety for you, then I suggest that you *substitute* them or choose some shorter, lighter routines for a few days. Prolonged stress can result in a compromised immune system, and getting sick is the last thing you would want to occur when you are already feeling as though you don't have enough time or energy to handle all your daily endeavors.

Lack of Time

Ever have one of those days when you somehow oversleep and the rest of your day feels as though you never got on track and had enough time? It's that feeling of wishing you had 3 extra hours in your day to get everything done. Well, that reaction could definitely affect your attitude and motivation to get your morning routine under your belt.

If you simply do not have enough time to run through your routine as you normally would, try squeezing it in, in bits and pieces. Many Pilates exercises can be adapted to standing positions. For example, while on the phone in the office, you could try a few repetitions of a standing version of the single-leg kick, or you could do a spine twist while seated in your office chair. There is nothing wrong with editing your routine to match your life. If you don't have time for your whole routine, you can also add exercise to your day by taking the stairs or by parking your car a bit further away from the entrance door of the grocery store or office building.

Not completing your usual morning routine will require some extra discipline on your part to remember to "cut and paste" your routine into your day, not an easy task if you have a jam-packed schedule. However, the upside to this solution is that you will probably rerelease small amounts of endorphins which will keep you feeling energetically more even keel and may prevent you from reaching for sugar or caffeine at some point.

Consider choosing a 20-minute routine if you normally go for the 40-minute one, or perhaps do at least a 10-minute quickie with your favorites to avoid skipping the workout altogether and losing your regularity. You know you will be glad you did it!

Boredom

Occasionally, boredom can set in because of repetitiveness within your routine, which can lead to loss of enthusiasm and result in lack of motivation. If it's just that you are feeling dull about your regular practice, try altering your choices or mixing them up a bit, kind of like hitting the shuffle key on your CD player.

Choose a different workout combination (if using the suggestions in this book) or perhaps take a class from a certified instructor for a couple of days or a week. Try a DVD or video that has been recommended to you, or refer to the references at the back of this book. These days, you can probably even find an Internet site with live streaming video workouts. Think about your session as fun, not work. The best way to stay fit is to approach it with an attitude of fun or play so that it doesn't feel like hard work. This may seem difficult initially if you are usually at the high end of the scale of productivity (I know I get that way). However, I encourage you to lighten up occasionally. I am not asking you to change your basic nature, but just stop to smell the roses. We live in an all-or-nothing society, either going full throttle or living on the couch. To stay healthy and fit for the long haul, you will need to be flexible in adapting your exercise regimen.

Change in Lifestyle

Sometimes a change in your lifestyle can also trip you up and catapult you into the trench of decreased motivation. Changing jobs, moving house, relocating to a new town, giving birth, getting married, acquiring a new ready-made family, or recovering from severe emotional shock (difficult illness, death in the family) all can decrease your motivation because of the large amounts of energy you expend adjusting to your new way of life.

Designing your routine to fit your current mental state can be another mind–body approach: You have to stick with a regular schedule yet adapt to immediate demands that may be distracting your focus from the exercise schedule. For example, if you are perhaps involved in a situation that is new, such as a new job position, or if you move to a different city, you might like to focus on choosing exercises in the routine that are particularly demanding in strength or coordination.

When challenged with a new lifestyle situation, the lack of familiarity and routine can throw you off your center. Performing exercises that are particularly challenging to your strength, flexibility, and coordination may just give you that extra boost of self-confidence if you can correlate the exercises to your particular personal situation.

For example, say you are hired as the new manger of a company, and the old manager was very well respected and liked. By choosing a routine that has some familiar exercises (you were hired because of your experience) but also some that challenge you in strength (e.g., front support with push-ups) and flexibility (e.g., spine stretch) and coordination (e.g., twist), you might find you have a sense of accomplishment, which in turn may assist you in feeling more empowered and confident in your new position. Remember, this is mind–body exercise, and that relationship goes well beyond the obvious.

Lack of Results

Everyone wants to know how long will it take to see results of Pilates exercise. The answer is, immediately. If you stand up straighter, engage your abdominals to tighten your midsection, straighten your shoulders, and hold your head up, you can immediately look so much better. Realistically, however, it may take anywhere from 5 to 10 sessions before you see a change in your body. Joe Pilates' saying was that in 10 sessions you feel different, in 20 sessions you see a difference, and in 30 sessions others notice the changes.

Pilates pays off for people who show the greatest patience. This is definitely a system where harder or faster is *not* better. Even those individuals who are quite fit should start at the foundation level. My teacher taught me that to learn this work correctly, you must approach it as though you were building a skyscraper. The foundation must be laid with care and allowed to set before you start building the structure taller and higher. If you build too high, too soon, your penthouse is going to wobble! We live in a rushed world where we want everything immediately, but Pilates works gradually.

If you have unrealistic expectations about the type of results you want and you fall short, de-motivation could rear its ugly head and you may unknowingly start to lose your positive, disciplined attitude. This is the time when seeking outside support might prove helpful. Your workout buddy might be able to offer some support just by listening. Many times you simply need an ear to hear you, and your workout partner might also be able to offer some insight into what might be contributing to your temporary lack of motivation. A Pilates professional may be able to assist you in reassessing your strengths and weaknesses, as well as offer you guidance in creating realistic goals. You may be unaware of something about your alignment or technique that might be influencing your ability to achieve your fitness goals, so a professional can offer an outside, experienced perspective. If you don't have contact with such a professional, you can always e-mail me through my Web site, www.synergypilates.com.

Genetics and age are two important factors over which you don't have a lot of say. You can thank your biological mother and father for influencing your body weight and muscle fiber composition. Body composition can greatly influence the way in which your musculature develops as well as performs. This factor in turn could affect your skill with Pilates routines, and if they are not up to your expectations, it could affect your level of motivation.

As for the age factor, well, what can I say: Time affects all of us and simply does not stop. Natural parts of the aging process include decrease in muscle tissue, loss of flexibility, stiffening of the spine and joints, decrease in metabolism, decrease in oxygen supply to muscles, and bone loss. These factors tend to creep in slowly, so you may not notice them in one day. Generally, you tend to start feeling that fatigue sets in sooner during your workout or you are not recovering as quickly when you finish. This process might cause some distress because it may lead to a lower level of expected results and therefore a loss in motivation.

But wait—it's not all bad news! Diet, sleep habits, stress reduction, workout commitment, and your particular regimen are huge factors over which you *are* well in control. By making intelligent choices you are able to contribute a lot to the formula of your health and wellness program. Construct your health habits wisely, intelligently, and realistically; and use outside professional guidance when you need someone's objective insight. The path to a well-balanced, healthy lifestyle is well within your grasp.

If You Just Don't Want To

We all have the days when we just don't feel like exercising. Creating some awareness around that lack of motivation is helpful. If you are truly exhausted both mentally (lack of sleep or rest, high level of stress) and physically (extremely sore and stiff muscles, pained or even slightly swollen joints), it's okay to skip your workout. Perhaps just going for a nice pleasure walk instead for about 15 to 30 minutes could help. No exact distance, no extreme hills, no goals—just a nice, easy pace to get your body moving, your circulation going, and your mind clear. If you are lucky enough to live near a beach or another natural type of setting, moving your body in nature and gazing at the ocean or trees can be invigorating and nurturing. Even if your nature walk is in your neighborhood, perhaps if you set your mental focus on noticing the trees, the sounds of birds, or even the way that your neighbors are designing their yards, your mind can enter a more relaxed state.

The important thing is that you have made the effort to get your body up and moving, which is the first step in getting your mental drive back on track. Taking a day off to refresh yourself so that you can return to your regular workout feeling renewed and motivated will most certainly give you the mental and physical rejuvenation you need to get back on the mat tomorrow.

Power of Positive Attitude

Trusting and believing in your own ability to achieve whatever it is you set your mind to is so important, not only for your physical fitness but for your mental health and well-being. As Joe Pilates said, "Physical fitness can neither be acquired by wishful thinking nor by outright purchase" (Pilates and Miller 1998, 6).

I don't know how many times I've had new clients come in for their first session only to immediately tell me what they *know* they "can't do," that they "don't have any abdominal muscles," or they "must be the most uncoordinated person you know." It makes me sad that these individuals have such a negative self-image and that by repeating their self-deprecating thought patterns, they are reinforcing these beliefs that limit their potential. In the studio, I have witnessed clients transform themselves through their belief in themselves, their dedication, and discipline. From overcoming a painful setback through injury, to emerging from childbirth with a completely different body and then working to regain the body's original capabilities, to dealing with genetic circumstances that limit physical capabilities, I have seen and applauded countless situations where it has been obvious that through the simple yet limitless potential of mental power, the human being has no boundaries. Many of us spend most of our time trying to control the things in our lives that we *can't* possibly control, but we forget that we *can* have nearly complete control over our own bodies and minds.

To gain this kind of control, you must commit to achieving your goals. This physical and mental commitment is probably the most important step on your road to empowerment. No one will wave a magic wand to suddenly make you fit, sexy, and rich. You have to work to accomplish your own goals. After all, once you experience success, no one will be more pleased than you!

2

Training Room Adjustments

||||||||||||||||||||||||||||||||||||||||||||||||||||||||||||||||||||||||||||||||||||||||||||||||||||||||||||||||||||||||||||||

If you exercise regularly at home, having your own private workout area is a must. The beauty of the Pilates method is that you do not need a lot of space or fancy equipment to do your workout. What you *do* need in your quest for continued workout adherence is the consistent regularity you create for yourself each day as well as a set space in which to exercise each morning.

The body and mind respond well to routine and regularity, and they respond even better when the actual environment has routine, or similarity, as well. So, not only do what you think (concentrating on your exercises and their execution) and do (performing the exercises themselves) have an impact on your success, but so does the very place where you choose to put yourself when you are working out. In this chapter, I share with you tips and ideas on your workout area itself, whether to choose a mat or exercise directly on the carpet, what sorts of props you might consider incorporating, functional workout wear, and ideas on how to stay focused on your workout routine.

Your Workout Space

Creating and using your own workout space is crucial to maintaining and enjoying your regular routine at home. Establishing a place to call your own for the time you have dedicated to your own regimen sends the message to yourself that *you*—and your efforts—are indeed important. Among the factors vital to a pleasant workout area are space, lighting, temperature, ventilation, cleanliness, and order.

- **Space to move.** If you have a separate room that you can dedicate solely to exercising, you are without a doubt very fortunate. If you don't have a separate room for your Pilates routines, you should establish a designated area. Perhaps a corner of your family room or living room might work nicely. Avoid using your bedroom if possible. Bedrooms are for resting and sleeping. After choosing a room, make sure it is free of clutter. To be sure that you have enough room to exercise without knocking anything over with your limbs, lie on the floor and make a snow angel. The feeling tone of Pilates is length and expansiveness, which you cannot accomplish if you set yourself up in an area that is too cramped and potentially injurious.

- **Lighting.** Lighting is important in creating the correct ambience in any room setting, your workout space included. For those of you arising and working out before the day breaks, it is extremely important to choose good lighting. Consider using full-spectrum lighting, which closely emulates natural sunlight. Light also leads to improved plant growth—maybe you can add some greenery to your workout space for extra oxygen!

- **Temperature.** Keep the room at a comfortable temperature. So for some of you who naturally feel colder, this may mean keeping it a bit warmer. My home workout space is shared with my office space. In the winter, I add to the room a small space heater that is plugged into a timer set to warm up the room about 30 minutes before I know I will be using it. This takes the chill out of the air and helps me stay on schedule with my home routine. If necessary, I leave the heater on to keep my muscles warm while I am working out and to prevent a chill when I am cooling down.

  For those of you who naturally feel hotter, keeping the room cooler or cracking the window, even in the warmer months, might be an option. Just be sure that you do not become chilled, especially if you tend to perspire freely. Cool air on warm skin with a bit of perspiration might feel temporarily good, but in the long run is not a good idea for muscles. With Pilates, you generally do not sweat profusely, but occasionally the weather may be warm, you might blast through without stopping to increase intensity, or you might choose a more challenging routine.

- **Ventilation.** You already know that the Pilates method is based on the principle of the breath and the breathing mechanism. So, it certainly makes sense to have optimal ventilation and air flow so that your effort to breathe with the optimal technique is enhanced with full, clean, fresh, and oxygenated air. You know how great it feels to breathe when you take a walk through a lush, green forest; when you spend a clear, brisk day at the beach; or when you go outside after a big rainstorm? That's because the air is filled with negative ions. Negative ions are odorless, tasteless, and invisible molecules that you inhale in abundance in certain environments. Think of mountains, waterfalls, and beaches. Once they reach the bloodstream, negative ions are believed to produce biochemical reactions that increase levels of the mood chemical serotonin, helping to relieve stress and boost your daytime energy.

According to Pierce J. Howard, PhD, author of *The Owner's Manual for the Brain: Everyday Applications from Mind-Brain Research* and director of research at the Center for Applied Cognitive Sciences in Charlotte, North Carolina, negative ions increase the flow of oxygen to the brain, resulting in higher alertness, decreased drowsiness, and more mental energy (2006) –all components of a productive morning workout. They also may protect against germs in the air, resulting in decreased irritation from inhaling various particles that make you sneeze, cough, or experience throat irritation. These symptoms are common to people who have pets or other allergies.

So, be sure to crack the windows when you can to allow fresh outside air to flow into your workout space. Of course, if weather or outside temperature does not allow for it, look into purchasing an air purifier or air ionizer. I have one in my home as well as in my studio, and I love the way they work.

• **Workout surface.** Now, let's actually get down to it—literally! I am talking about the floor underneath you, of course. It definitely should be adequately padded so that your spine and pelvis are not bruised. Many of the Pilates exercises have you on your back rolling through your spinal column or on your front with your hip bones pressed into the floor. My first choice is a carpeted surface that is quite firm with a dense, padded mat. However, your workout area may have hardwood or tile flooring, so you may need an extra-thick mat. Many types of mats are on the market today. They range from mats specifically designed for Pilates to basic yoga sticky mats that vary in thickness from 1/16 to 1/4 inch (1/4 to 1/2 centimeter). Type of firmness will range from extremely firm to quite spongy. It really is a personal preference, so you may need to experiment. If you can afford it, having a couple of choices might be the option for you. You could keep one type of mat handy for home use and a thinner, lighter-weight mat for travel. When I go on the road, I travel with an extremely thin, lightweight yoga travel mat that I can fold or roll up easily into my suitcase and use on top of carpet (usually in a hotel room) or, if staying with a friend who has hardwood floors, I use it with a thick towel on top of it.

Speaking of towels, some of you may prefer just to throw a large beach towel down on your carpet and not bother with anything extra. Some of you may even just exercise directly on top of the carpet; if you tend to perspire, it may not be the most ideal choice. I do not recommend using only a towel on a hard surface. You will probably bruise yourself, not to mention a towel will tend to slide on tile or hardwood flooring. Whatever type of surface you end up with, be sure it works for you so that you are not thinking about your mat more than your workout!

- **Music.** If you like to have music to work out to, setting up a small stereo or MP3 player with a speaker might be ideal for you. Wearing headphones is not practical because the wiring is cumbersome and distracting. When I trained in London at the Alan Herdman Studio, we always had music playing in the background. Usually something classical or occasionally some opera. I generally use music in my mat classes; classical, trance (but not too draggy), and world groove usually work for me. I avoid music with vocals as I find vocals disruptive and competitive with my vocal instruction in the class, but of course, unless you are talking to yourself out loud during your workout, it will probably not be a factor for you. I like to have music playing simply to fill up the background but definitely not to keep a beat to. Purists may say that music is a distraction and that the breath itself should be the inner music you attune your body to. Try both and see what works best for you. You may find that some days you wish to have it and other days you don't.

- **Decor.** If you are among the lucky and have a permanent workout space, decorate it in a manner that is as pleasant for you as possible. Perhaps you have some posters of fitness heroes or heroines (even yourself!) or photographs of nature that give you a sense of tuning within and being mindful. What better place to hang them for inspiration than on the walls of your personal workout sanctuary.

Painting the room an uplifting color might be another way to keep your energy active and moving for your workout. I can attest for this one: When I changed the color scheme at my studio from subdued lavender to a livelier goldenrod yellow, the impact of color was undeniably apparent. Everyone, including both my trainers and clients, was invigorated—just by the color! Additionally, if you get up very early and live in an area where the sun is not always streaming through the window, a lighter color on the walls plus appropriate additional lighting could factor into maintaining your level of inspiration.

You can see some effort is involved in establishing a supportive and aesthetically pleasing yet productive personal workout space. I firmly believe that the time and energy you put into creating the most positive environment will not only give you creative satisfaction but will also reward you with the feeling of anticipation of your daily appointment with yourself. On top of that, with those two factors going for you, the physical return you will achieve from your efforts will more than reward you for all that you have chosen to undertake.

Props and Workout Aids

Props can be used to adjust the difficulty of an exercise. Prop use can make an exercise less challenging or accommodate for various limitations. For those of you who are ultrafit, props can be used to create variations to refresh your regular routine. The following list includes some inexpensive props you might want to help you keep your routines safe, challenging, and creative. I suggest keeping them in a small basket or workout bag that can be tucked neatly away when not in use.

- **Strength bands.** It is best to have one heavy and one medium band. Strength bands can be used to assist in stretching when the leg muscles are tight and to enhance strength movements. They can also be used for respiratory strengthening by placing a band flat around the lower ribs and using it for tactile feedback to feel posterior lateral (back and side) rib cage breathing. They are handy for travel as well.

- **Small red rubber Mikasa ball.** A 500 millimeter ball is appropriate. Mikasa balls are useful as a prop to assist with inner thigh awareness on exercises when you wish to keep the legs parallel. Simply place a ball between the ankles or slightly above the knees.

- **Dowel.** It should be about 1/2 inch (1.3 centimeters) in diameter and 3 feet long (1 meter). Dowels can be very helpful when extending the arms alongside the ears or in front of the chest to optimize arm placement.

- **Small hand towel.** Use a small hand towel by placing underneath the back or side of the head to keep the neck in a comfortably aligned position. They are also handy if you start to perspire.

- **Single tennis ball.** Single tennis balls offer a myriad of possibilities. Use between the ankles or above the knees to keep legs parallel; stand on one and massage the bottom of your foot; or lie on your back and roll it around underneath your middle back or a tight hip or buttock. They are travel friendly.

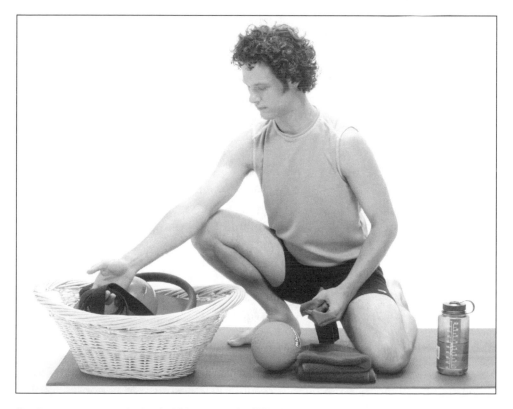

Keeping your props organized and within easy reach will keep you on track with your morning exercise routine.

- **Two tennis balls taped together.** The tennis balls can also be enclosed in an old tube sock. This is useful, again, at the ankle or upper knee to engage the inner thighs and is easier than a Mikasa ball or single tennis ball. When placed so that the balls lie on either side of the spine, it can be used to massage the muscles along the spine. This too is easy to pack in a suitcase.

- **Pilates Magic Circle.** The Magic Circle can be used between the hands similar to how you would hold a dowel. Additionally, placed between the ankles or above the inside of the knees, it will help keep you mindful of your inner thighs. If you have a Magic Circle with padding on the inside, you can place the circle so it is outside the ankles or upper knees and engage the outer hip muscles.

- **Small pillow or cushion.** These are always useful to have in case you need some extra padding underneath your knees or head.

- **Fitness ball.** Choose a fitness ball according to your height: 55 centimeters (for those shorter than 5 feet 7 inches), 65 centimeters (for those 5 feet 7 inches to about 6 feet), and 75 centimeter (for those 6 feet and taller). When you sit on a ball that is the correct size, both your hip and knee joints will be at 90-degree angles.

Whether or not you occasionally use media to stay inspired is up to you. So many DVDs and videos are available these days that it can be daunting. Because this book is designed to keep you inspired on your own with options for creating different routines, you may or may not opt to have a television with a DVD player nearby. It will also depend on where your workout area is located. A study, den, family room, office, or a living room, is likely to have a television and DVD player. Where the screen is located relative to your being able to see it from the floor might be problematic. Be sure to have the screen situated in a position that you are able to view it without having to contort yourself, which could potentially become a distraction.

If you are working out in a room that does not have media readily available but you have a laptop computer, you may wish to use it with DVDs. You might also be able to play live streaming exercise videos from your computer. If you find that you enjoy the convenience and occasional stimulation of using an instructional video but your workout space is located where media options are not available, consider purchasing a small television with a DVD player attached; this equipment is widely available and is usually not outrageously expensive. You will have to determine whether the investment will be worth it to you in the long run.

Clothing

With workout clothing now being a multibillion-dollar industry, you will not have a shortage to choose from. Everyone from top designers to discount stores is getting on the fitness clothing bandwagon. I suggest that you choose clothing that is comfortable yet practical. You can choose from leggings, tank tops, shorts, sweatpants, sport tops, and T-shirts. If you are not used to formfitting exercise wear, you may feel that you need to hide your body initially, but clothing that allows you to see what parts of you are working will be best. Additionally, formfitting clothing will allow you to be more aware of your alignment as your kinesthetic awareness increases, an all-important skill you will develop as you continue your adherence to your workout routines.

If you tend to perspire readily, clothing made with moisture-wicking material may be a more comfortable choice for you. This material includes polypropylene and other synthetic blends. While 100 percent cotton feels good against the skin, once it is wet from perspiration, it tends to feel heavy and you could get chilled toward the end when you are stretching or lying in your rest pose.

As you become more and more adept at the routines, you will be able to sail through them more quickly and may begin to perspire a bit more freely. Be sure to not allow your body and muscles to become chilled; it could cause extra stiffness later. I prefer layering because I tend to get cold easily. For the top, I usually wear a sleeveless base layer followed by a thinner, long-sleeved T-shirt, and perhaps a medium-weight sweatshirt on top. For the bottom half, I like to wear leggings or boot-cut bottoms that are fitted through the hips and thighs, and I avoid waistbands and seams that might exert unnecessary pressure on sensitive areas of the body. While baggy bottoms may initially seem more comfortable, they can conceal your pelvis and legs, thus hindering your placement awareness.

Many people like to wear socks when they do their Pilates routines. While socks keep your feet a little bit warmer, the feet slip inside of the socks when working on a sticky mat or carpet. If you must wear socks, a great choice is called Toesox (www.toesox.com). These fabulous socks are the creation of Joe Patterson and are made from the perfect cotton–Lycra blend so that each toe has its own fitted covering. In addition, the bottom of the sole is covered with tiny rubber dots that prevent the foot from slipping. They are a great choice for keeping your feet warm (but not uncomfortably warm) as well as anchoring your feet in place to avoid slipping when holding some of the plank positions or downward dog. I wear these in my studio, especially in the colder months, and my trainers and clients love them.

3

Muscles Into Action

||||||||||||||||||||||||||||||||||||||||||||||||||||||||||||||||||||||||||||||||||||||||||||||||||||||||||||||||||||||||||||||||||||

Many of you are already very aware that the Pilates method can contribute to good posture. However, you may not be aware of how posture affects how your muscles work and, consequently, your ability to execute the exercises for optimal results. Posture and the position of your muscles during your workout also affect your ability to breathe (*the* Pilates fundamental). And, because you have chosen the morning as your preferred workout time, warming up the muscles correctly to avoid injury and soreness and understanding how to synergistically connect to your Pilates core are extremely important. It sets the tone for the rest of your waking hours.

For those of you who are newer to Pilates, the information in this chapter is essential to building a foundation of skill and correct movement. This understanding helps you gain the most from your efforts. For readers who consider themselves proficient and experienced with this work, I encourage you to read this chapter as well. It will deepen your understanding of Pilates and give you a chance to assess your current technique and perhaps even enhance it. So, sit up straight, take a deep breath, and get ready to understand how your body moves and works.

Alignment: Stacking It Up

Good posture goes with you wherever you go and in whatever position you might be. To get the most out of your workout, you need to know about postural lines through the body. Why does this matter? Because the Pilates method relies on alignment for its effectiveness. When you perform minimal repetitions, each one counts for efficiency and effectiveness. In addition, misalignment (through injury, habit, poor postural awareness, or muscular imbalances) increases the risk of injury. Posture and alignment dictate your movement: Poor posture results in poor movement mechanics; good posture results in better movement mechanics. Pilates *can and will* improve your posture and your awareness of it. So, let me share with you some alignment basics to enable you to assess your current condition.

Start out facing a full-length mirror. Stand with your feet pointing straight ahead and the inside edges approximately one of your own foot's width apart. From the front, your chin, the notch in between your collarbones, your navel, and the middle of your pubic bone should be aligned straight up and down. As for your legs, ideally, the middle of your hip joint (*not* your hip bone), middle of your kneecap, tibial tuberosity (the bony protrusion at the top of your shinbone below the knee), and second toe should make another straight line. (See figure 3.1.)

Now turn to the side. You may need someone to take a photo of you so that your head can face forward and you can assess your head and neck placement. Your earlobe, the acromion process (bone that juts out on the top of the shoulder area), lateral torso line, greater trochanter (larger bony protrusion at the top of your outer thigh), lateral knee joint, down to just in front of the lateral ankle bone all should make another straight line. (See figure 3.2.)

Now you definitely will need some assistance, unless you have a situation where you have mirrors set up so that you have a clear view of your entire back body from head to toe. Look for a straight line from the base of the skull, through the center of the spinal column and down through the tailbone to a midpoint between both feet. With the legs, look for a straight line from the sit bones down through the middle of each heel. (See figure 3.3.)

These lines are called plumb lines and are indicative of skeletal alignment (or misalignment, as the case may be). They intersect bony landmarks, skeletal points that are easier to see and that help determine whether any discrepancies are occurring. Body alignment is a good indicator of muscle function. Your muscles are designed to create efficient and effective movement if the structure on which the muscles rest is positioned (aligned) correctly. Skeletal charts include these plumb lines, so you can use them to observe how the bones should be stacked up. Remember, gravity is always pulling downward, so if the bones are not stacked up, compensation occurs at the next juncture.

To extend the idea of stacking, picture a stack of kids' building blocks. If one block is situated too far to one side, the next one on top has to be positioned far to the opposite side to prevent the whole structure from tumbling down. Although humans are not made of blocks, the body will automatically, but unknowingly

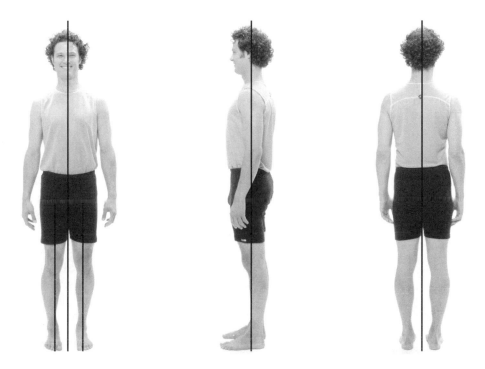

FIGURE 3.1   Proper postural alignment, anterior view.

FIGURE 3.2   Proper postural alignment, lateral view.

FIGURE 3.3   Proper postural alignment, posterior view.

compensate for misalignment; and what happens then is that muscles do not work as they are meant to, which results in perhaps the wrong muscles taking over to do a movement. This cycle continues over time until one day the body is injured due to excessive joint wear and tear that can lead to arthritis or other problems, and poor movement mechanics.

The pelvic girdle and shoulder girdle placements, along with the spine and diaphragm, are major players in understanding posture as well as truly learning how to strengthen the core. The pelvic girdle's positioning directly influences the curvature of the lumbar spine, and it is the point where the legs connect to the torso. The shoulder girdle positioning significantly influences the alignment of the head and neck as well as the arms' movement mechanics.

Pelvic Girdle

The pelvic girdle is the Grand Central Station of the trunk where ground forces from below (impact from walking) meet the compression of the weight of the upper trunk and its movements. It is where all forces are distributed and transferred. Ideally, your pelvis is in what is known as neutral pelvic alignment. This is to say, your hipbones are in the same vertical plane as your pubic bone. With your pelvis in this alignment, your hip sockets will be as neutral as possible and so will your lumbar spine. "Neutral" simply means the positioning of the bones are such that the muscles can function optimally and joint impact is minimized.

The position of your pelvis is crucial for the muscles of the hip joint and legs to function optimally. This position will influence your ability to perform most of the Pilates mat exercises to get maximum benefits with minimal risk of injury. Furthermore, because pelvic alignment directly influences the lumbar spine, understanding how to get and keep your pelvis in neutral position is extremely important. Some people have pelvic girdles that aren't neutrally aligned; instead they have anterior or posterior tilts.

Anterior Pelvic Tilt When you have an anterior tilt of the pelvis, your hip bones are in front of your pubic bone and your low-back (lumbar) area is much more concave and arched (lumbar lordosis; see figure 3.4). The muscles in your lower back are short and tight, the vertebral column is compressed in back (which means the vertebrae are squashing your discs—*not* a good thing), and the abdominal muscles are long and weak. Also, the hip flexors are short and tight, and the hip joint is in chronic flexion (compressed). For example, when you attempt an exercise such

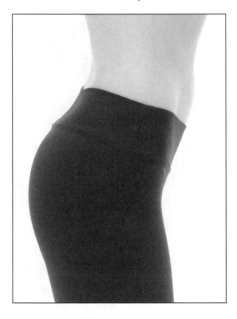

as the rollover, the tightness of the lower back hinders you in your attempt to round the lower back to bring the legs overhead smoothly. In the double-leg kick, the tight hip flexors inhibit your ability to use the correct muscles to lift your legs up, making you recruit your low-back muscles instead (not efficient, and potentially injurious).

If you have determined that you have an anterior tilt, specifically focus on the lunge stretches to stretch the hip flexors, which contribute to that particular misalignment. Particularly avoid arching your lower back more when you are in the lunge stretch position. When the hip flexors hit their end range and you attempt to go further, *more* anterior pelvic tilt can occur in your attempt to stretch further. That result is not what you are looking for!

FIGURE 3.4 Anterior pelvic tilt.

Posterior Pelvic Tilt When you have a posterior tilt of the pelvis, you find your hip bones behind your pubic bone and your lower back convex, or flattened to the rear of you (see figure 3.5). The lower back structures (muscles, tendons, bones) are chronically stressed, and the hamstrings are usually short and tight. The hip flexors become long and weak, and the hip joint in chronic extension can create irritation because the head of the thigh bone (femur) is putting constant pressure against the front upper portion of the hip socket. With a posterior tilt, when you attempt to do any of the Pilates exercises that require you to be in a seated upright position (spine stretch, spine spiral, saw), the tightness of your hamstrings, which is preventing you from sitting up in neutral position, causes undue strain on the lower back.

If you have determined that you have a posterior tilt, focus on stretching your hamstrings, paying particular attention to maintaining a neutral pelvis when doing so. The origin of the hamstrings is at your sit bones, and they go down and insert well below the knee. So, you feel the stretch all along the entire back line of your leg, perhaps feeling it more in one particular segment of the hamstring than another. Be sure to keep the knee straight but not locked, keep the ankle flexed at the heel, and avoid hiking up one side of the hip (usually the stretching side).

Either pelvic misalignment causes undue strain on the lumbar vertebrae and hip sockets, and it will affect the mechanics of your entire body. Guiding the physical structure, starting with the pelvis back to neutral is most important in order to reap the most benefit from the Pilates method and your morning workouts.

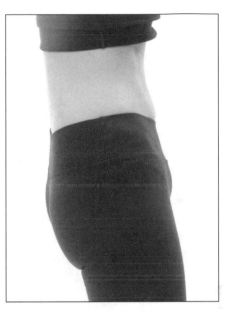

FIGURE 3.5   Posterior pelvic tilt.

Shoulder Girdle

If you have a collapsed chest with rounded shoulders (typical for people who sit a lot at their jobs), your middle and upper back will be convex to the rear, a condition called kyphosis. Many times with this misalignment, the shoulder blades (scapulae) are placed too far to the side of the upper back (abducted) affecting your ability to properly move your arms. When your shoulder joints are restricted, you will "borrow" the movement from your lower spine or your neck. Because a fair amount of Pilates exercises require the arms to move through and beyond these ranges, this alignment is something that needs to be addressed.

Another unwanted result of this shoulder and upper back misalignment is a forward-placed head (see figure 3.6). This position causes excessive compression on the vertebrae in the back of the neck and weakens the muscles in the front of the neck. Excessive compression is never a good thing to have occurring in the spinal

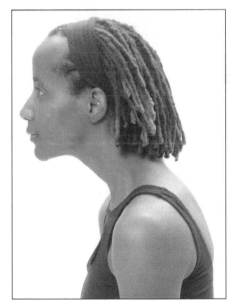

FIGURE 3.6   Forward-placed head.

column or in the neck. It can adversely affect nerves that lead to your shoulders, elbows, wrists, and hands. Here are two types of shoulder misalignments and exercises to correct them so that your shoulder girdle is in great shape for your Pilates workouts.

Rounded Shoulders With the rounded shoulder, collapsed chest, hunchback upper torso, you must incorporate specific stretches for the front of the shoulders and chest. Additionally, you should be aware of your head and neck placement. Some shoulder openers exist within the workouts themselves (see roll-up with strength band, seated shoulder stretch), but I also suggest supplementing with additional time devoted to opening this area, especially if you are aware of it affecting your posture.

To stretch the chest, stand in a doorway with the arms out like the letter T and with the elbows bent at 90 degrees. Place the elbows on one side of the door frame with the forearms perpendicular to the upper arm. Gently lean the upper torso forward, moving the chest through the doorway. Be very careful to avoid thrusting your head forward or overarching your lower back. You should feel a gentle stretch across the upper chest and shoulders. Some of you who are very tight might also feel some stretching across the top of the shoulders as well. Hold this position for at least a minute or so. This is a great stretch because it can be done nearly anywhere, even at work.

To work on the forward-head misalignment, an easy exercise is to stand and place your hand on your nose. Slowly bring the head back and slightly up on a diagonal, as though your chin is reaching back and up toward the base of your skull. Your head will move back anywhere from 1 to a few inches (at least 3 centimeters). Notice how far back you have moved your head. The distance from where your hand is after you move your head back, is how far forward your head has been. Keep your head in place, and feel the position. Note how you probably feel your abdominals working a little bit more. See if you can carry this head placement awareness throughout the day and check yourself periodically.

Arched Back If, on the other hand, you have perhaps had a lot of gymnastics, dance, or military training, your middle and upper back will be quite flattened or even arched so that the chest juts forward. This type of upper body placement causes excessive tightness along the entire spine, especially the middle and lower back. This tightness can then potentially adversely affect the ability of the diaphragm to move fully, thus your breathing is not at its fullest or best (an issue with the rounded shoulder alignment as well). This situation is not good, because Pilates relies on breathing as a primary way of connecting with the deep abdominals. Rigidity in the rib cage also contributes to poor breathing mechanics, another result of this misalignment.

One simple way to start to regain the curvature in the upper and middle back is to practice breathing in the all-fours, hands-and-knees position. Start with the hands placed directly under the shoulders and the knees under the hips. As much as possible, keep the spine neutral. Inhale, and as you exhale, slowly curve the spine toward the ceiling into a cat position (spine convex to the ceiling), strongly using the abdominals to facilitate the movement. Tuck the head under, gazing toward your thighs with the pelvis tucked under, tailbone drawn toward the head. Holding this position, breathe in deeply and gently work to curve the spine more into the assumed position. Additionally, envision your shoulder blades widening on your back with the in breath as well. Your inhalation helps to curve the upper thoracic spine more into its ideal position (convex to the back). Breathe in this position for a few breaths, and then slowly return back to the starting position.

So you can see that either position of the upper torso and shoulder girdle can cause undue strain in the upper back and neck, affect the movement mechanics of the arms, create excessive neck and shoulder tension, as well as affect your respiratory ability. I cannot emphasize enough how important this is, because good quality breathing is the golden key to the Pilates method.

The Core and the Inner Unit

"Core" seems to have become the buzzword as of late. You might hear someone with back pain say, "I know I need to strengthen my core." Or you might hear, "My doctor has recommended that I start core-strengthening exercises." Well, what exactly *is* the core? The average person gestures toward middle and points to the abdominal area. This answer is partially correct.

The core is the lumbopelvic and hip complex, where the body's center of gravity is located and from where all movement is navigated. The inner unit consists of four muscles: the diaphragm, the transversus abdominis, the multifidus, and the pelvic floor. Collectively, they form a corset around the lumbar spine and pelvis, a flexible cylinder of support with a top and a bottom that enables safe movement. The inner unit is the main component of the core.

The lumbopelvic hip complex is not the only part of the body that needs stabilization. In the upper torso, the shoulder blades also need stabilization for the arms to move on the torso without unnecessarily disturbing the spine, head, and neck. Additionally, muscles surrounding the shoulder joint and shoulder blade areas may need some strengthening and stretching for proper arm movement to occur. In this chapter I offer you some preliminary exercises before the workouts themselves so that you might better isolate and create a clearer awareness of these crucial four muscles. Once your kinesthetic awareness is such that you are very aware of your four core muscles working together, not only do you avoid injury, but you gain an even deeper level of benefit from the workouts themselves.

In the Pilates method all movements originate from the core, so it is important to understand how to connect to these important stabilizers. The benefits of training the inner unit are many and are interconnected. But before we get to connecting them together as a team, it is imperative that you be aware of them individually in isolation, because they usually tend to be weak and challenging to "feel." Because form and alignment are the key ingredients of good movement, and good movement is also a by-product of mental focus, the skills of coordination and timing will be developed. This will enable you to become deeply aware of joint positioning (proprioception), which is necessary for optimal neuromuscular repatterning (teaching your brain to do the same movement through a different nervous pathway). Strengthening and repatterning of the neuromuscular system develops strength and stability in the four core components. Dynamic stability within a gravitation field is what ends up developing; and that is what you need all day long whether you are sitting, standing, or walking!

Diaphragm

The diaphragm is perhaps the most important member of the inner unit, as it is the primary muscle used in respiration. If you have been involved with the Pilates system of exercise for a while, you are very aware of how all movements seem to have a specific breath pattern to them. The ability to adapt your breath to whatever you are calling it to do is called respiratory control, which requires respiratory strength as well as the skills of coordination and timing. As you develop your breathing skills, you can then enhance your workout with specific respiratory musculature strengthening.

Another important aspect of a strong respiratory system is that with each breath, you can decompress the discs in your spine and become taller! Becoming taller allows you to move more freely through the spine. When one inhales properly, the ribs in the thoracic or middle spine rotate to assist the diaphragm in its descent, rotating the rib head at its attachment to the vertebra and, similar to a crowbar's movement, it opens the space where each vertebral disc lies! Thus with breath alone, axial lengthening (an increase in length along the spinal line of the torso) of the spinal column occurs—a spinal adjustment with no appointment and no fee!

Maintaining as much disc space as possible keeps your spine young. Your discs are similar to sponges. With each movement they are slightly compressed and then rebound back to hopefully their original, plumped-up, or less compressed state. When they rebound, they draw moisture from the tissue surrounding them, thus they are nourished and hydrated. In the book *Return to Life Through Contrology*, Joe Pilates said, "If your spine is inflexibly stiff at 30, you are old; if it is completely flexible at 60, you are young" (Pilates and Miller 1998, 16).

It is obvious that a lengthened, healthy, and supple spine will help you move more freely through your Pilates routines. To optimize the respiratory system, the diaphragm, which is the primary breathing muscle, must be aligned over the pelvic floor. For optimal breathing to occur, physiologically efficient alignment must be in place. No slumping, no slouching! (i.e., shoulder girdle over a neutral pelvic girdle with spinal curvatures intact and not deviated). Thus, alignment supports breath and breath supports alignment.

The bottom surface of the lungs sits on the top surface of the diaphragm. Thus, when the diaphragm contracts and moves down, it pulls on the lungs and by negative pressure, air is pushed into the lungs (inhalation). When the diaphragm relaxes, it moves upward. The volume of the lungs decreases, and air is expelled (exhalation). This event is approximately 1.5 centimeters in its ascent and descent during normal breathing at rest. It can increase to as much as 7 centimeters during deep breathing (Ganong 2005). The important event of breathing can occur with this much capacity only when your posture is aligned.

Breathing into the posterior lateral (back and side) portion of the trunk is specific to the Pilates method. In my studio we refer to breathing as "the golden key." With good breathing skills, you enhance the effectiveness of your workout and more fully oxygenate your blood. Also, with the healthy ascent and descent of the diaphragm, your internal organs get a massage. Joe Pilates termed this an "internal shower." In his book *Return to Life Through Contrology,* he teaches that to breathe correctly, you must completely inhale and exhale, always working very hard to "squeeze" every atom of impure air from your lungs in much the same manner that you would wring every drop of water from a wet cloth. This "internal shower," or internal wringing out, also stimulates the management of your lymph glands, which assist your circulatory system (Pilates and Miller 1998).

Classic Pilates breathing is in through the nose and out through the mouth. However, studies show that nostril breathing does not only give you deeper and fuller breaths, it directs those breaths to the lower lobes of the lungs where maximum oxygen exchange takes place—the very reason you need to breathe! Nose breathing also signals the body to release hormones associated with pleasure and a sense of calm, such as beta-endorphins. Conversely, mouth breathing stimulates the release of fight-or-flight stress hormones and causes the ribs and chest to become inflexible (Douillard 2001). Thus, I teach nostril breathing to my clients. I find that for some it feels natural right away and others have to adjust to it over time. Experiment to find what seems to work best for you, but consider the information you have learned here. You may become convinced to breathe in and out through your nose.

The diaphragm is unlike any other muscle in the body in that it inserts on its own central tendon, not on any bone or other external structure. To keep this discussion simple: The diaphragm is a dome-shaped structure having contact with the middle and lower ribs where it has a relationship to the transversus abdominis, with the breastbone, and then to root-shaped structures that run alongside the lumbar vertebrae. It is very much like an opened umbrella shape that, through the movement of the ribs, pulls on the tissue at the bottom of the lungs, thus forcing air to be pulled in.

I would like to offer you some specifics on how to focus solely on feeling the breath. This focus is vital to your technique in performing the workouts in this book, because the cylinder of strength that you develop in your core starts with this breathing skill to get in touch with the correct way to engage the deep pelvic and lumbar stabilizers.

In a seated position, either on a chair or on the floor with the legs crossed, place your hands in a horseshoe shape at the base of the ribs. Your thumb will be at the back floating ribs, and sides of your index fingers will be at the bottom of the ribs in the front. Sit as upright as you can. Take an inhalation through your nose, directing it toward your thumbs in the back of your body. Feel the expansion of the lower ribs in all directions.

As you breathe out, feel your ribs come together and specifically "funnel" them together, especially in the front, as though you want them to make a funnel right down *inside* the front waistband of your pants. Just by creating this action, you will be activating your transversus abdominis, which is also a part of the inner unit. Once you have fully exhaled, and you feel the ribs have funneled, work to keep them that way as you take your subsequent next inhale. Do not become rigid or stiffen the torso, but avoid pushing the abdominal wall outward to take your inhalation. It is a good idea to watch yourself in a mirror initially so that you avoid elevating your shoulders when you practice. For now, avoid taking breaths that are abnormally long and excessive so that you can isolate the correct respiratory muscles.

Transversus Abdominis

The transversus abdominis, also referred to as the TA, is the innermost abdominal muscle that connects to the spine at the back through connective tissue and wraps around the trunk to meet its counterpart in the front. You can feel the TA on the lower abdomen just inside the hip bones. When this muscle contracts it causes a slight narrowing of the waist and a flattening of the lower abdomen (but *not* navel to spine—more on that later!). It functions to "stiffen" the vertebrae of the spine and stabilize the pelvis prior to movements of the arms, legs, and torso. It does this by generating a pull on the connective tissue (fascia) upon engaging. The contraction generated is a pull and is subtle in sensation. It is *not* a feeling of hollowing or scooping, but the feeling of tension resulting from engaging the tissues. The sensation of contraction is always less than you usually think it ought to be! In people who use proper stabilization and recruitment technique, the TA is frequently active at a low level throughout the day.

Eventually, you will need to be able to recruit this muscle in many different positions such as side-lying, seated, standing, on hands and knees, facedown (prone), and face up (supine). For now, focus on finding it in the face up position. One of the easiest ways I have found for individuals to find and feel this muscle is through a prolonged exhalation. Place the pads of your index and middle fingers on the most prominent parts of your hip bones, then move them toward your navel approximately 1.5 inches (4 centimeters). Lie on your back with your knees bent, feet flat on the floor. Take a breath in, and exhale slowly and steadily until your fingers feel as though they are being absorbed by the abdominal region. Avoid forcing the muscle to contract. Because the TA is one of the primary respiratory muscles for expelling air from the body, it automatically contracts. If the lower abdomen bulges or pushes outward, a different muscle is being activated and chances are you have unknowingly substituted the obliques. Again, remember that the contraction is probably a lot less in sensation than you think it should be. Look for a feeling of the tissue pulling apart or spreading out and flattening. You can use the image of pulling plastic wrap over a bowl.

Correct recruitment of the TA is crucial for engaging the deep abdominal wall and effectively learning how to stabilize the pelvis. Without efficient usage of this important part of your inner unit, you miss one of the most important pieces of the Pilates method and you flirt with injury. To effectively train the TA, follow these principles:

- Ensure that the initial contraction is isolated (and no other muscles are being substituted).
- Begin the contraction slowly and with control.
- Exert low effort.
- Breathe normally.
- Never squeeze the buttocks or flatten the lower spine to the floor to feel this muscle working.
- Never bulge out of the abdominal area as you are working.

Isolation of the TA is a part of neuromuscular repatterning. It is a process, not an event; just as life is about the journey, not the destination. So, in other words: Train slowly with focus, intention, and awareness so that the development of this skill is reinforced with all your subsequent exercise or movement choices.

Even experienced Pilates participants, including some of my colleagues, do not correctly recruit their TA. Do not be discouraged if at first you find you have been substituting your obliques or rectus abdominis all along. Try connecting to your TA at various times during your nonexercising moments such as while driving a car, standing in line at the grocery store, sitting and chatting on the phone. It will help you to become more aware of it in conscious action so that it becomes strong and available to you unconsciously as well.

Multifidus

The multifidus is a very deep back muscle. It is part of the erector spinae group, which is located right along the vertebrae in the middle of the spine and on the posterior surface of the sacrum (a wedge-shaped bone in the back of the pelvic girdle). It is contained within an envelope of connective tissue. This connective tissue, called fascia, tightens when the multifidus contracts. This increased tension braces the posterior pelvis, and together with the transversus abdominis is the third component of the inner unit.

In Pilates we are most concerned with the sacral portion of the multifidus. For the sacral multifidus to fire, the sacrum must be positioned correctly. This means the sacrum must sit in between the two back pelvic bones (ilium) with the top, which is actually called the sacral base (the wedge shape is like an arrow pointing down), slightly angled forward and the pelvis in neutral, neither in an anterior nor posterior tilt. *If the pelvis is not in neutral position, absolutely, the sacral multifidus will not fire, and you will not have the support on the back side of the pelvic girdle from this very important part of the inner unit.* The sacral multifidus is extremely challenging to feel when it is working, so I hope to assist you in finding and connecting with it.

Try the following:

1. From a upright seated position, see in your mind's eye a point of reference at the back of your navel and the other at the top (base) of your sacrum (a midpoint between your two sacroiliac joints (the two bony points you can feel on either side of the sacral base). Feel your weight evenly distributed between both sit bones side to side, as well as front to back. Now, as you breathe out and connect to your TA, imagine drawing the back of the navel toward the sacral base and the sacral base toward the back of your navel. Do not allow yourself to actually move any of your skeletal structure. See whether you can be aware of a tingling type of sensation on your sacrum and maybe even up your spine. This is your multifidus gently engaging.

2. Start again sitting upright with your weight evenly distributed on the sit bones as in the previous description. Imagine someone grasping the back of your waistband and giving it a slow pull upward (as though you were getting goosed!). Again, *avoid any skeletal compensatory movement.* Once again, the sensation you feel along your spine, especially in your sacral area, is your multifidus.

This muscle does not contract the way you normally are used to feeling a muscle contract. It does not harden underneath your touch. If you were to actually palpate the sacrum by gently resting your fingers on the surface, you may feel the tissue there "swelling" or "puffing up." When one palpates the surface of the sacrum and it is contracting, it feels under the fingertips like a perfectly ripe avocado when you are testing it for ripeness. Remember, this muscle in particular is the most challenging to locate and become aware of, so don't get frustrated if you do not connect to it right away.

Pelvic Floor

Your pelvic floor consists of a hammock of musculature that connects the pubic bone at the front to the tailbone and sit bones at the back. Three muscles make up the pelvic floor, but for our intention here, we are primarily interested in connecting to the portion closest to the front and nearest the pubic bone because it directly relates to deepening your connection to the TA. The pelvic floor is considered the diaphragm of the pelvis and may be compared to being the bottom lid of the cylinder of the inner unit. The top of the cylinder would be the diaphragm itself, while the TA and multifidus comprise the actual cylindrical portion. In Pilates exercises, the alignment of the two diaphragms is crucial for optimal function and performance in alignment, breathing, stability, and movement.

The pelvic floor functions to support and control the internal organs. Remember, when you inhale, the diaphragm lowers and displaces the internal organs downward pressing on the pelvic floor. Therefore, this musculature must be resilient enough to accommodate the weight of the organs descending with an inhale and also to "spring" back when you exhale. The pelvic floor supports all movement through its fascial connection to the TA and needs to have both strength and flexibility.

The individual pelvic floor muscles must be balanced in their function to properly stabilize your core. So, not only must you become aware of and be able to connect to the pelvic floor, you should be able to work toward specifically connecting with the anterior (front) portion. Why? Without going too deeply into anatomy, the answer is that the anterior (front) position is fascially connected to the TA. When you fire the anterior pelvic floor, you deepen the contraction of the TA. When you overengage the posterior (back) position of your pelvic floor, the buttocks and rectum engage and you most likely tilt the pelvis into a posterior position, thus losing your neutral pelvic alignment and misaligning the sacrum. This causes the multifidus to lose the ability to fire and support the back of the sacrum. To reap the benefits of the inner unit and therefore *all* of the Pilates exercises, all four components of the inner unit need to work synergistically together.

To specifically work on strengthening your neuromuscular connection to the pelvic floor, try this exercise: Start in a seated upright position either on the floor or a chair. Visualize the pelvic floor as a diamond shaped trampoline connecting the tailbone to the right sit bone, and the right sit bone to the right side of your public bone. Then connect the tailbone to the left sit bone, and the left sit bone to the left side of your public bone. These four points anchor your pelvic trampoline. Inhale to prepare, and upon exhaling imagine bringing this trampoline upward as though you have jumped in the center of it and it is rebounding you upward. You have to actively recruit these muscles, and one of the most common instructions on how to do so is to contract and hold the muscles you would use to stop the stream of urination. After you have become aware of the sensation of connecting to your pelvic floor, work to hold your connection for longer lengths of time—initially just contracting the muscle for 1 to 5 seconds and building up to 10 to 20 seconds. Be sure you are breathing while holding the connection!

You now know how to feel and connect to your TA, and you know how these two components of your inner unit are related. Now, go back to the exercise where you isolate the sensation of connecting to your TA using the breath (see page 36), and add in the pelvic trampoline action so that the two areas are working simultaneously. As your awareness of and strength in these two areas increase, you will begin to notice how one stimulates, or fires, the other. This very specific connection is something that will develop in strength and skill over time, and it is not without a challenge. However, if you practice, it can be done, and your reward will be a much deeper and integrated connection to your inner unit and a safer more effective workout.

Although challenging, the beauty of strengthening the pelvic floor is that it can be done anywhere, anytime—and no one will ever know you are exercising! In fact, I encourage you to work to strengthen the pelvic floor as much as possible during your day. Whether you are standing in line at the grocery store, sitting in your car in traffic, going for a walk, or exercising with this book; the more you practice contracting this muscle, the stronger it will quickly become. And, you will not only notice the contraction and connection to the pelvic floor, you will become more aware of its relationship to and stimulation of the TA as well. This awareness is vital to enhancing the workout benefits of your Pilates exercise routines.

Relationship Between Alignment and Inner Unit

Now you know the effect that alignment and the inner unit have on your workout, and you know how to tap into each to enhance your workout and maximize your potential. However, one question remains: How do alignment and the inner unit work together? When both are optimized, you can reach a whole new level of efficiency and effectiveness from your morning workouts. Optimal postural alignment allows for the most favorable conditions in which to train for neuromuscular efficiency (i.e., how well the brain communicates instructions to the muscles through the nervous system). The dynamic stability of your postural alignment (whether you are still or moving against gravity) allows the body to compensate for the effects of gravity, ground reaction forces, and momentum at the right joint, in the right plane, at the right time (coordination and timing). For example, think of being able to catch yourself from falling if you step off a sidewalk curb and accidentally catch your foot and trip.

The core musculature is an integral piece of a protective mechanism that relieves the spine of potential injurious compression during movement and activities. The goals of core stability training are to increase strength and muscular endurance of the lumbopelvic hip complex and optimize neuromuscular control. Greater neuromuscular control and stabilization strength lead to a more biomechanically efficient posture. I said it before, and I will say it again: Posture and alignment dictate movement. An inefficient neuromuscular system will cause you to substitute the inappropriate muscles for movement, which can lead to poor movement, potential injury, and worsened bad postural habits.

Warming Up

Now that you are in alignment, in touch with your core, breathing as optimally as possible, and are aware of how to move your body in synergy, let's get going with your pre-Pilates warm-up! Most of us do not leap out of bed ready to launch into an all-out workout. This is the time of day when our minds are much clearer, but our bodies may feel just a bit stiffer. Thus, some rhythmic movements to raise core body temperature, lubricate the joints, and just plain old rev up the circulation might be a good thing.

Benefits of a gentle warm-up include the following:

- It warms your muscles by increasing the movement of blood through your tissues, making the muscles more supple.

- It increases delivery of oxygen and nutrients to your muscles by increasing the blood flow to them.
- It prepares your muscles for stretching.
- It prepares your heart for an increase in activity.
- It prepares you mentally for the upcoming exercise.
- It primes your nerve-to-muscle pathways to be ready for exercise.

To warm up for Pilates exercise, any of these choices would be great; you could even interchange them as you work to keep your workout fresh and challenging: marching in place, jumping on a rebounder or mini trampoline, making a few revolutions on a stationary bike, taking a brisk walk around the block (the fresh air is an added bonus), jumping rope, good old-fashioned aerobic class type movements, or yoga sun salutations. We all tend to get into habitual routine, but choosing a different warm-up each time could keep you motivated as well as help to burn a few extra calories.

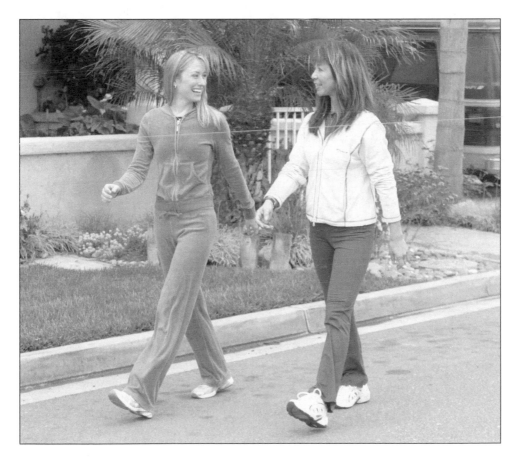

A warm-up fitness walk with a workout buddy can add variety to your routine and keep you motivated.

I encourage you to warm up for a minimum of 5 minutes before beginning your routine of choice. If you happen to feel especially stiff on some mornings, a slightly longer warm-up at a lower level of intensity might be a better choice than a shorter warm-up at a higher level of intensity. This suggestion is wise if you are especially sore as well. Obviously, how much time you have for your routine and your warm-up will be a factor if your schedule is tight. Be sure to choose your warm-up and Pilates routine accordingly to avoid having to stop without a proper stretch when you finish.

No one warm-up is more beneficial than another in the morning, but remember that *warming up* is exactly that and must be done starting at a lower level of intensity and then moving gently upward. Be sure that it gets all your major joints (spine, ankles and feet, knees and hips, shoulders, arms, and neck) moving through their range of motion as well as raises your core body temperature. You should be able to feel your temperature rise.

Of course if you have the luxury of a longer warm-up, or perhaps you incorporate some sort of cardiovascular exercise as part of your fully faceted exercise regimen, you may choose to go for that long run or bike ride before your Pilates routine. If so, be sure to adequately cool down a bit before you start your mat exercises. If you have perspired quite heavily, change into some dry clothes so that your muscles don't get chilled. If your hair and scalp have gotten damp, towel dry as much as possible. You already know about the importance of hydration—you lose fluid even without exercise. So, consider drinking a glass of water before starting your Pilates routine, and keep some nearby for sipping during your workout.

Adaptation is a well-known phenomenon in the exercise world. It means that if you do the same routine the same way, in the same order, at the same pace, and so on, your body adapts and soon learns how to expend the least amount of energy for the same amount of work. Your mind is less stimulated as well. Significant improvements in performance occur when the appropriate exercise stresses are introduced into your training program. So I suggest you vary the type of warm-up you do at least every couple of weeks to keep your body and mind from getting bored.

What To Do When You Overdo It

While you do want to feel that you have exercised, you should feel exhilarated after a workout. When done correctly, exercise should leave you with increased mental and physical energy. However, you may occasionally experience some muscle pain or soreness. If you are changing your routine by increasing intensity or duration, or if you are getting back into shape again after a little layoff, you can expect to experience some muscle soreness. Muscular discomfort occurs normally about 24 to 48 hours after your workout. The best response to it is to continue with a slightly modified routine and some additional stretching.

To modify your routine, I suggest choosing a slightly longer warm-up with a slightly less intense Pilates routine (e.g., either lighter in intensity or shorter in duration or both) for a day or two. Be sure to drink plenty of water to help flush out the lactic acid build-up (a chemical by-product of exercising that gets stored in the muscles) that can also contribute to excessive soreness. Taking a hot shower before and after your workout, a hot bath in Epsom salt, and indulging in a massage treatment can also be beneficial in easing muscle soreness.

At times pain or discomfort is more troublesome and indicative of a more serious problem. Here are some general guidelines from Dr. Cedric Bryant, Chief Exercise Physiologist for the American Council on Exercise (Bryant 2005), that can help you determine whether or not the pain you are experiencing warrants a cessation of exercise or medical attention.

- **Joint pain or discomfort.** Joint pain of any degree of severity should not be ignored. Pain in the ankle, knee, elbow, or wrist is especially concerning; these joints are not covered by muscles, so the pain is rarely muscle related.
- **Localized pain or discomfort.** If the pain occurs at a specific location, it is likely an early indicator of some type of injury. If the pain does not occur in the same location on the opposite side of the body, consult a doctor.
- **Persistent pain or discomfort.** If the pain persists for longer than 2 weeks or gets worse, see a health care professional. It is especially important if the pain does not respond to standard methods of treatment (e.g., rest, ice, over-the-counter pain medications).
- **Swelling in or around the area of pain.** Swelling is a classic sign of an injury and should never be ignored. It is not uncommon for swelling in or around a joint to cause pain and stiffness.
- **Your normal routine is disturbed.** Pain that interrupts your sleep patterns or interferes with work or normal daily activities is a strong indication of a more serious problem.

In general, avoid pushing through or working through pain. The "no pain, no gain" saying is outdated, inaccurate, and unsafe. Pain is the body's way of communicating to you that a problem exists and an injury may be on the horizon. Your ability to discern the mental and physical state of your body is another step in the journey to total mind–body awareness.

part two

Workouts By Time and Intensity

 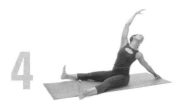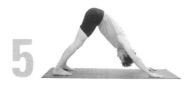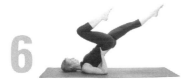

4

Light Workouts

20-Minute Light Workout

The 20-minute light workout is a great place to start if you are a bit newer to the Pilates technique, you are just getting back into a routine after illness or another break from exercise, or it's just one of those days when you don't have a lot of time or mental energy to push yourself harder. This routine will give you just enough in terms of spinal articulation, abdominal and back strengthening, as well as challenge your legs and upper body. Do this routine when you just don't feel like it. You will be glad you did.

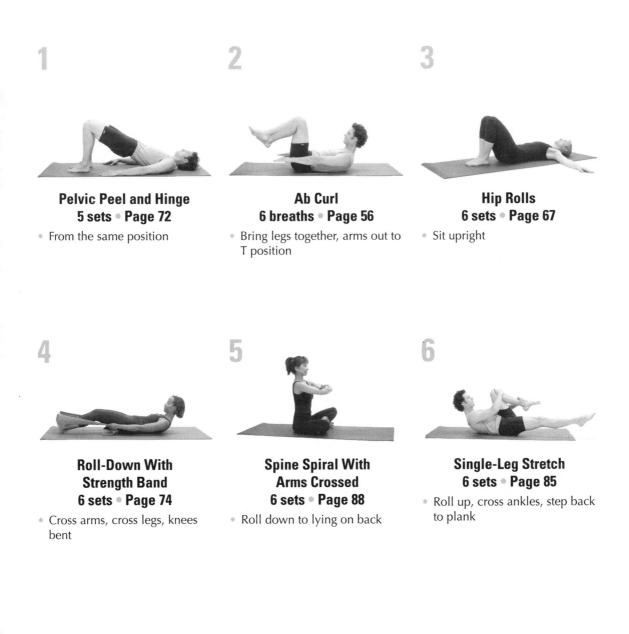

1

Pelvic Peel and Hinge
5 sets • Page 72

- From the same position

2

Ab Curl
6 breaths • Page 56

- Bring legs together, arms out to T position

3

Hip Rolls
6 sets • Page 67

- Sit upright

4

Roll-Down With Strength Band
6 sets • Page 74

- Cross arms, cross legs, knees bent

5

Spine Spiral With Arms Crossed
6 sets • Page 88

- Roll down to lying on back

6

Single-Leg Stretch
6 sets • Page 85

- Roll up, cross ankles, step back to plank

7

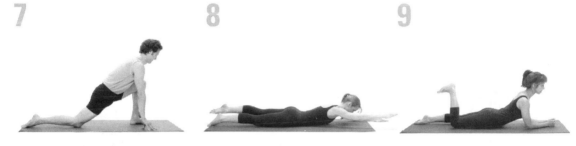

**Lunge With Hands and
Knee on Floor
1 minute per side • Page 70**

• Step to plank, lower to floor

8

**Slow Swim
5 sets • Page 87**

• Come up to bent-elbow cobra

9

**Single-Leg Kick
6 sets • Page 84**

• Hands and knees to modified
plank

10

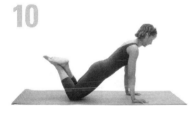

**Knee Push-Up
5 to 10 sets • Page 68**

• Sit back

11

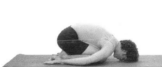

**Child's Pose
30 to 60 seconds • Page 59**

40-Minute Light Workout

The 40-minute light workout is for those of you who have now built up some endurance, stamina, and strength to go twice as long as the 20-minute light routine. It is also perfect for those of you who have been exercising regularly but may be a bit fatigued from lack of sleep, outside stresses, travel, or illness. Perhaps you have been overdoing it lately and still wish to keep up your regularity but need to back off a bit in terms of intensity. This routine challenges your ability to control your body at a deeper level by incorporating more balance (rolling, balance rocker) and timing (coordination, seated abduction and adduction).

1

2

3

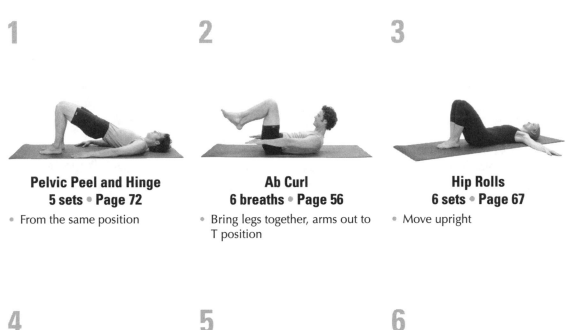

Pelvic Peel and Hinge
5 sets • Page 72
- From the same position

Ab Curl
6 breaths • Page 56
- Bring legs together, arms out to T position

Hip Rolls
6 sets • Page 67
- Move upright

4

5

6

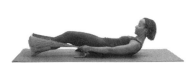

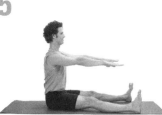

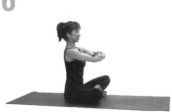

Roll-Down With
Strength Band
6 sets • Page 74
- Remain upright on last repetition

Spine Stretch
6 sets • Page 90
- From the same position

Spine Spiral With Arms
Crossed
6 sets • Page 88
- Place hands behind

7

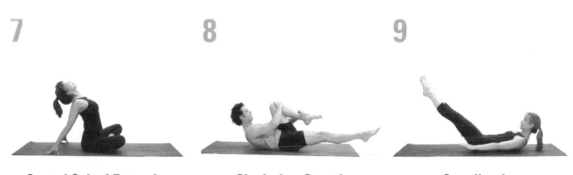

**Seated Spinal Extension
With Arm Support
5 breaths • Page 81**

- Roll down to floor

8

**Single-Leg Stretch
8 sets • Page 85**

- Legs to tabletop position, arms to ceiling

9

**Coordination
6 sets • Page 60**

- Roll up

10

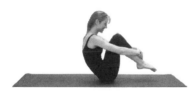

**Rolling
5 sets • Page 75**

- Straighten legs, grasp ankles

11

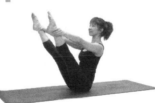

**Balance Rocker
5 breaths • Page 57**

- Bring legs to floor, open arms

12

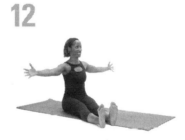

**Seated Abduction and
Adduction
6 sets • Page 79**

- Cross ankles, step back to plank

(continued)

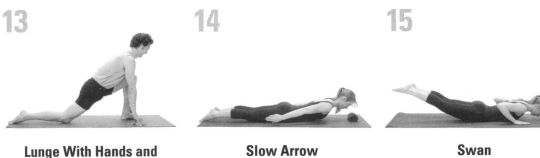

13

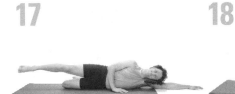

14

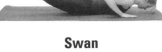

15

**Lunge With Hands and
Knee on Floor
30 seconds per leg
Page 70**

• Move to plank, lower to floor

**Slow Arrow
6 sets • Page 86**

• Bring hands flat near shoulders

**Swan
6 sets • Page 91**

• Come up to bent-elbow cobra

16

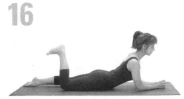

17

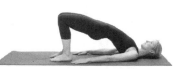

18

**Single-Leg Kick
6 sets • Page 84**

• Roll to one side

**Side Kick
8 sets • Page 83**

• Roll onto back

**Shoulder Bridge Hold
8 breaths • Page 82**

• From same position

19

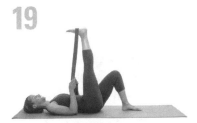

20

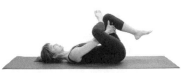

21

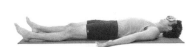

**Hamstring and Inner Thigh
Stretch With Band
Hold 30 to 60 seconds
Page 66**

• From same position

**Figure 4 Stretch
Hold 30 to 60 seconds
Page 63**

• From same position

**Corpse
Hold 3 minutes • Page 61**

The 60-minute light workout is designed for those of you who have been participating regularly and have the luxury of a full hour to devote to working out. The intensity level is still light, so again if you have been a little short on the shut-eye, are newer to a regular Pilates routine, or perhaps need to lighten the difficulty factor for a day, this workout is the choice for you. This routine is thorough and includes stretches that will leave you energized for the full day you have ahead of you!

1

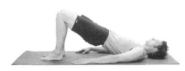

Pelvic Peel and Hinge
5 sets • Page 72

- From the same position

2

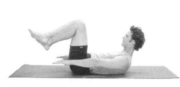

Ab Curl
6 breaths • Page 56

- Bring legs straight up to ceiling, arms in T position

3

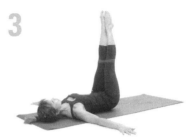

Pendulum
5 sets • Page 73

- Roll up to seated position

4

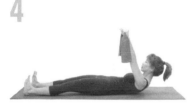

Roll-Up With Shoulder Rotation
8 sets • Page 77

- Remain upright on final repetition

5

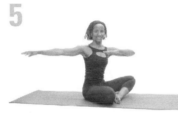

Spine Spiral With Elbow Extension
8 sets • Page 89

- From the same position

6

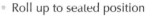
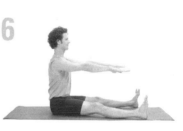

Spine Stretch
6 sets • Page 90

- Fold legs to chest, wrap arms around legs

7

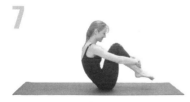

Rolling
6 sets • Page 75

- Open legs, bend knees, cradle calves

8

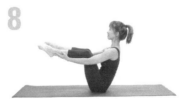

Half-Open Leg Rocker
6 sets • Page 65

- Lower legs open in V position, arms open

9

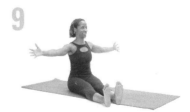

Seated Abduction and Adduction
6 sets • Page 79

- Legs together, roll down to floor

(continued)

10

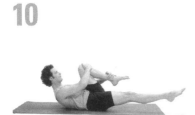

Single-Leg Stretch
8 sets • Page 85

* Bend knees to tabletop, arms to ceiling

11

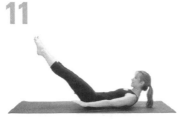

Coordination
8 sets • Page 60

* Lower legs to floor, arms at sides

12

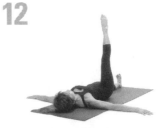

Leg Circles
5 circles each direction per leg • Page 69

* Roll up, cross ankles, move into plank

13

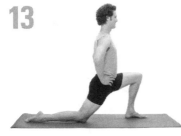

Lunge With Transitioning Torso
30 to 60 seconds per side
Page 71

* Lower torso to floor

14

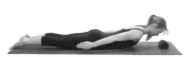

Slow Arrow
6 sets • Page 86

* Bend elbows, prop torso, bent-elbow cobra

15

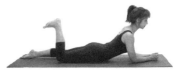

Single-Leg Kick
6 sets • Page 84

* Press to hands and knees

16

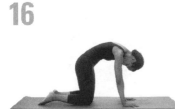

Cat Stretch
4 sets • Page 58

* Lie facedown on floor

17

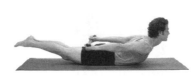

Double-Leg Kick With Strength Band
6 sets • Page 62

* Press to hands and knees

18

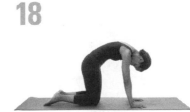

Cat Stretch
2 sets • Page 58

* Lie facedown on floor

19

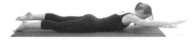

Slow Swim
8 sets • Page 87

- Hands and knees, to seated upright

20

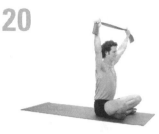

Seated Shoulder Stretch
6 sets • Page 80

- Cross ankles, bend knees, move to plank

21

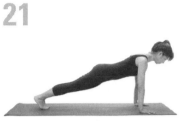

Front Support
6 breaths
5 sets leg pulses (optional)
Page 64

- Turn to lie on side

22

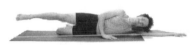

Side Kick
5 sets per side • Page 83

- Roll onto back

23

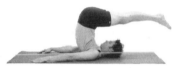

Rollover
4 sets legs open,
4 sets legs close • Page 76

- Bend knees, place feet flat on floor

24

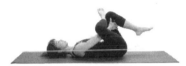

Figure 4 Stretch
30 to 60 seconds per leg
Page 63

- Stretch out both legs

25

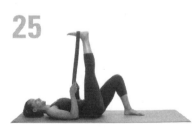

Hamstring and Inner Thigh Stretch With Band
30 seconds per stretch
per leg • Page 66

Ab Curl

Begin lying on your back, place your feet flat on the floor (1) or legs in the air with knees bent at 90-degree angles, ankles crossed, knees open above the hips. Bend the knees, and align the heels with the sit bones. Place the arms next to your trunk with the palms down. Put a small ball or rolled towel between the inner thighs. Inhale. As you exhale, bring the upper torso forward, hinging at the T point (located straight back to the spine from the lowest point of the breastbone), arms reaching toward the feet and hovering parallel to the floor (2). Breathe in for 3 counts, and breathe out for 4 counts for 6 complete cycles. Inhale for a seventh breath. As you exhale, slowly return the torso back to the starting position using the abdominals. Maintain a neutral pelvis during the entire exercise.

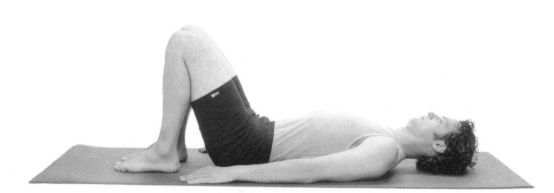

1

2

Balance Rocker

Begin balanced just behind the tailbone, keeping your legs straight and shoulder-distance apart and your hands grasping the top of the ankles (1). Arms are straight, toes are softly pointed, and the spine is slightly flexed. Inhale and exhale for 5 complete breaths. Engage the inner unit as well as the shoulder blade stabilizers to balance in this position. If hamstrings are an issue, bend the knees so that the shins are parallel to the floor and cradle the calves in your forearms (2).

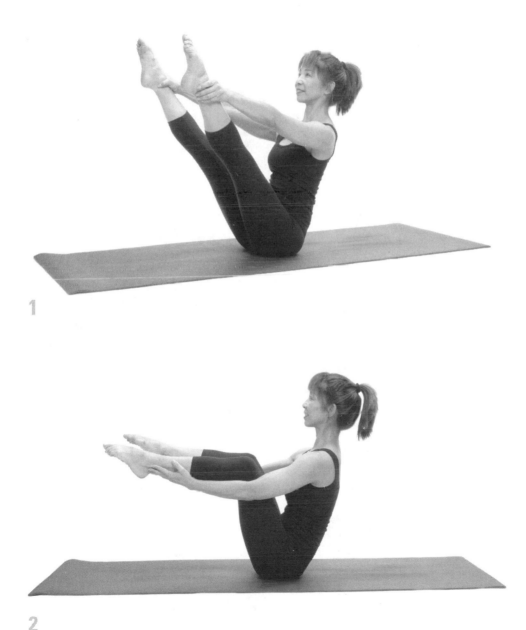

1

2

Cat Stretch

Begin in a quadruped position with the hands directly beneath the shoulders and the knees directly below the hips (1). Maintain a neutral pelvis and stabilized shoulder girdle. Align the head and neck with the rest of the spine. Inhale. As you exhale, begin to contract the deep abdominals and gently curve the spine into a convex arch so that the spine is flexed and curved toward the ceiling (2). Inhale. As you exhale, begin to articulate through the spinal column as you move from the flexed position to an extended, arched position (3). Avoid hunching the shoulders by using the scapulae stabilizers to draw the shoulder blades down the back whether in a flexed or extended spinal position. Allow the breath to carry the movement like a wave rippling through the spine. Avoid overworking. This movement is meant to alleviate any accumulated tension in the body. Repeat 4 or 5 sets.

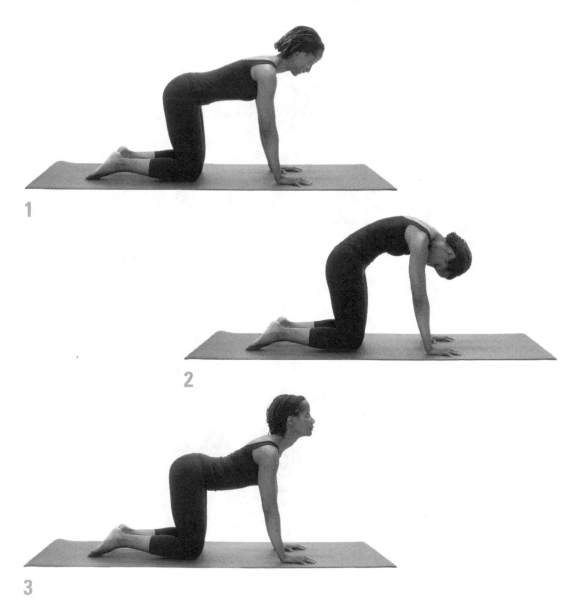

1

2

3

Child's Pose

Facing the floor, begin with your knees bent and buttocks on the heels and the thighs open so that the chest can rest on the legs. Place your arms either behind you, toward your buttocks with the palms up, or place them alongside the head with the palms down. If your buttocks do not rest on your heels, place a cushion or towel that is thick enough so that the buttocks will have something to rest on. Breathe normally in this position.

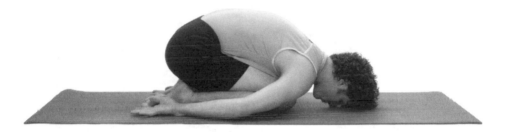

Coordination

Begin lying on your back with the knees bent, shins parallel to the floor, legs together, and toes softly pointed (1). Arms are straight and perpendicular to the floor. Inhale. As you exhale, simultaneously extend the legs forward to 45 degrees, lower the arms so that they hover near the hips, and curl the upper torso forward (2). Inhale as you open and close the legs no wider than the shoulders (3), exhale as you bend the knees back to the starting position, and return the upper torso to the floor (4).

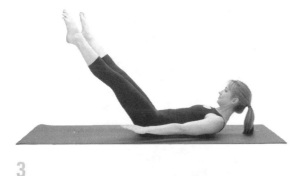

1

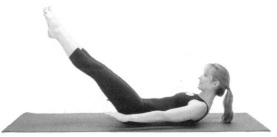

2

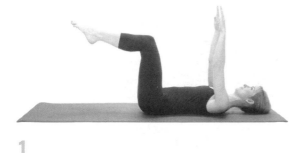

3

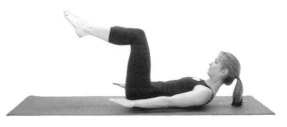

4

Corpse

Begin lying on your back with the arms out and away from the torso and the palms up. Position the legs slightly apart, and let them flop open. Close your eyes and mouth, and relax your jaw. With each progressive breath, allow your face to soften, the corners of your mouth to release, and the space between your eyebrows to open. Feel the tension drain from your body like grains of sands dribbling through an hourglass, slowly and steadily with each subsequent breath. Breathe deeply and completely and let go.

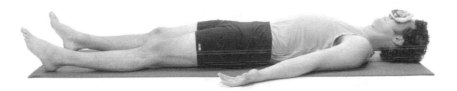

Double-Leg Kick With Strength Band

Lie facedown with the legs together, arms behind you, elbows bent, your hands at your lower back, grasping a strength band (1). Your hands should be at the width of your waist, and your elbows should be resting on the floor. Turn the head to one side. Engage the inner unit. As you inhale, bend the knees and pulse the feet toward the buttocks 3 times (2). As you exhale, stretch the arms out behind you with the palms facing inward, stretch the legs long and reach them away from you slightly off the floor, and extend (arch) the entire upper torso (3). Avoid overarching in the neck area. As you return to the starting position, turn your head in the opposite direction. As you inhale again, repeat the pulsing action of the feet toward the buttocks. Make sure your elbows are once again resting on the floor.

Note: Elbows may or may not be completely resting on the floor. Tight external rotator muscles of the shoulder girdle may inhibit this position. *Do not force elbows to the floor.*

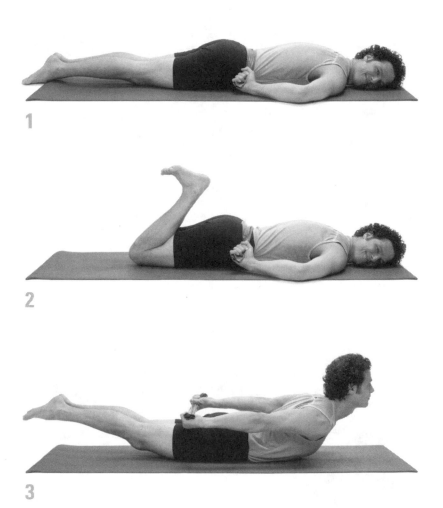

Figure 4 Stretch

Begin lying on your back with your right ankle crossed over the left leg just above the knee. Cross your right outer ankle bone so that it is to the outside of the left thigh with the right knee open to the right. Grasp the left thigh with both hands, and use your right elbow to press the right knee open to the right to increase the stretch. Keep your pelvis as neutral as possible. If your external hip rotators (those are what you are stretching) are too tight and you are unable to grasp your left thigh comfortably, use a strap around the thigh. Be sure to change sides after holding the first side a minimum of 30 seconds.

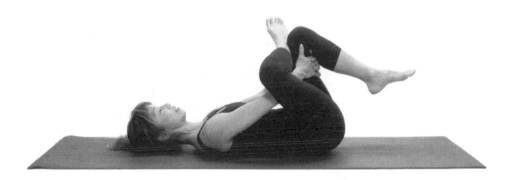

Front Support

Begin in a quadruped position (1). Bring the hips forward so that you support most of the body weight with your upper body. Your hips should be in one straight line with your head and neck, shoulders, and knees in a diagonal neutral position. You may as an alternative bend the knees and cross the ankles in the air or keep the shins and tops of the feet on the floor. Engage the scapulae stabilizers, the inner unit, and lower glutes. Maintain this position as you breathe in and out for six complete breaths. You can build up to ten breaths. Feel the workload distributed throughout the entire body. For an added challenge, you can add lep pulses (2). Inhale. As you exhale, pulse the entire leg up behind you 2 times only so far that you do not distort the line of the torso and supporting leg as well as the stability of the pelvis. As you inhale, lower the leg. Repeat again with the other leg.

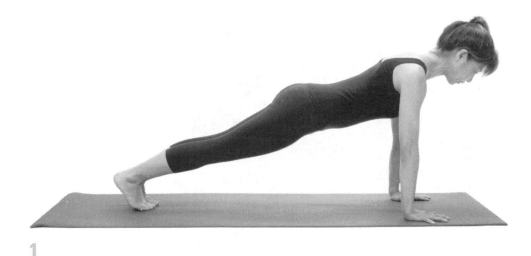

1

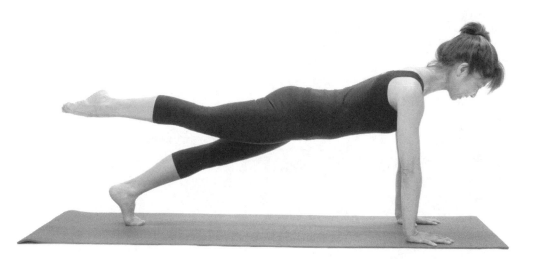

2

Half-Open Leg Rocker

Begin balanced just in front of the tailbone with the legs bent at the knees and shoulder-distance apart, the forearms or hands cradling the calves, and the shins parallel to the floor (1). Point the toes softly, and slightly flex the spine. Inhale, lengthening the spine. As you exhale, engage the abdominals to roll back to just the upper back (2). Continue exhaling to return to the starting position. The spine is slightly flexed to ensure even rolling. Use the abdominals (through the breath) as the impetus for rolling back, as well as to brake the upward movement to stop in the starting position. *Never roll onto the neck.*

This exercise is contraindicated for those individuals with thoracic osteoporosis or pre-existing neck issues.

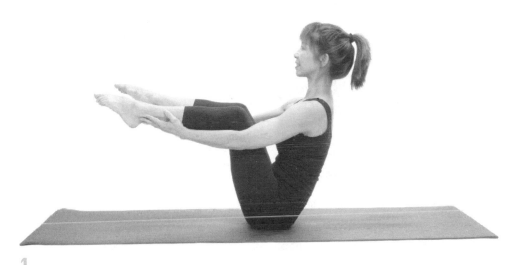

1

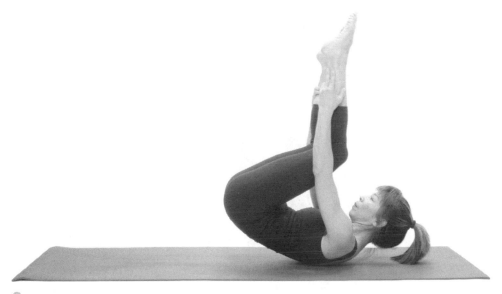

2

Hamstring and Inner Thigh Stretch With Band

Hamstrings: Begin lying on your back with the left leg bent and left foot flat on the floor (1). Extend the right leg to the ceiling, the ankle flexed with a strap, both hands grasping the ends of the strap, and the elbows placed on the floor. Anchor the pelvis in neutral. Hold the position for 30 to 60 seconds, and repeat with the other leg. *Inner Thigh*: Begin in the same position as for the hamstrings, but bring the leg to the outside of the torso avoiding any rocking to the side or hiking up of the pelvis (2). Hold the position for 30 to 60 seconds, and repeat with the other leg.

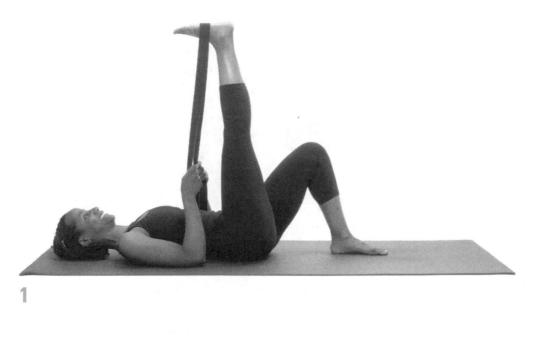

1

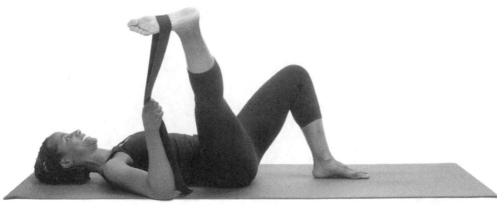

2

Hip Rolls

Lie on your back with your legs together and feet flat on the floor. Place your arms to the sides to form a letter T (1) or alongside the torso for more of a challenge. You may place a small pillow under your head for comfort. Inhale. As you exhale, roll the pelvis to one side, keeping the legs pressed together (2). Guide the rotation of the pelvis from the obliques, not by swinging the knees side to side. Inhale to bring the pelvis with the legs back to the starting position. Repeat to the other side. Be sure to keep the upper torso still. The head may rotate in the opposite direction from the knees if it doesn't strain the neck. Breath may be reversed to challenge respiratory strength.

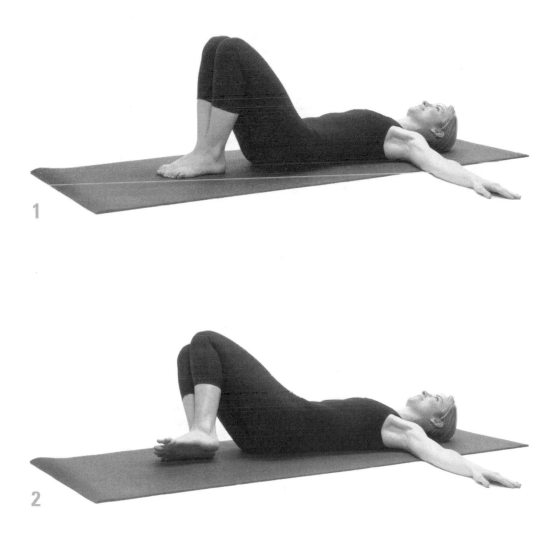

Knee Push-Up

Facing the floor, in a modified plank position, place the arms straight beneath the shoulders perpendicular to the floor (1). Bend the knees and cross the ankles. Form a straight, diagonal line with the head, neck, shoulders, pelvis, and knees. Inhale as you bend the elbows and lower the torso toward the floor (2). As you exhale, straighten the arms and return to the starting position. Distribute your work through the entire body, and be sure the pelvis is in neutral with the head and neck placement in line with the rest of your spine.

Option: Holding this position, breathe in and out for 5 to 10 full breaths.

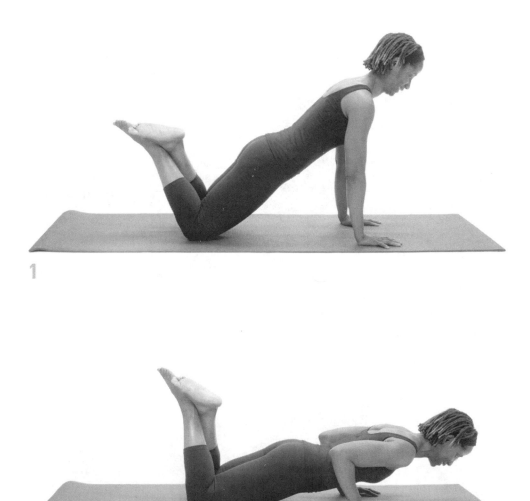

1

2

Leg Circles

Lie on your back with one leg on the floor with the ankle flexed and the other leg reaching to the ceiling, perpendicular to the hip socket, with the foot softly pointed (1). Position the arms to form a letter T, or alongside the torso for more of a challenge. Inhale and exhale one sequence as you anchor the inner unit and pelvis securely in place. As you inhale again, bring the leg in the air slightly across the midline of the torso, keeping the rest of the body stable (2). Exhaling, continue circling the leg down away from you (3), slightly out to the side (4), and back to the starting position. Circle the leg 5 times from the inside and 5 times from the outside. Be sure to keep the pelvis securely anchored in position as the leg rotates in the socket. If the hamstrings are tight, bend the knee of the moving leg. If you feel strain in the lower back, bend the knee of the resting leg, and keep the foot flat on the floor.

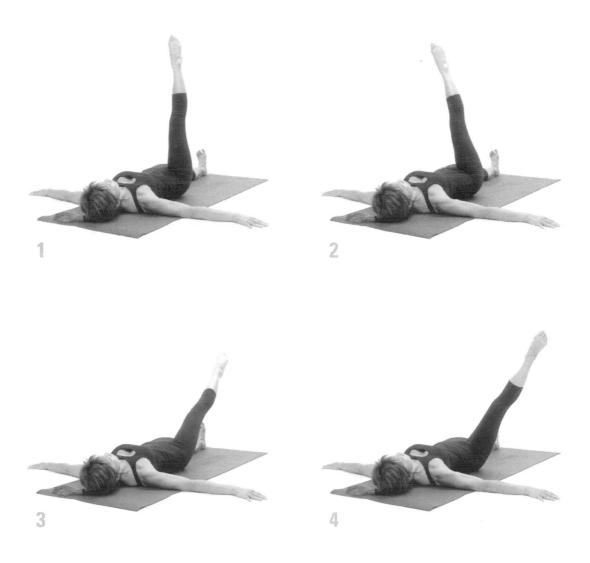

Lunge With Hands and Knee on Floor

From a kneeling position, bring one foot forward and keep other leg behind you. Lunge the torso forward until you feel a stretch in the back leg in the front of the hip joint and top of that thigh. Place hands on either side of the front foot. Keep the back knee down with the top of the foot toward the floor. Hold this position to stretch the hip flexors and upper thigh (quadriceps). Be sure to keep your pelvis level with both hip bones square to the front of your mat. Change sides. Inner unit on!

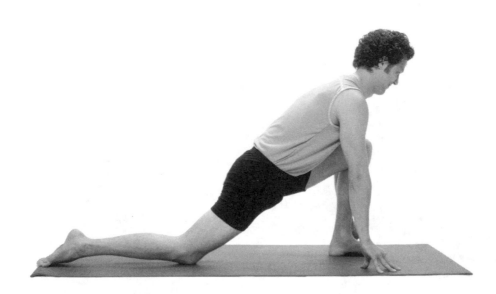

Lunge With Transitioning Torso

From a kneeling position, bring one foot forward and keep other leg behind you (1). Lunge the torso forward until you feel a stretch in the back leg in the front of the hip joint and top of that thigh. Place the hands on either side of the front foot. Keep the back knee down with the top of the foot toward the floor. Hold this position to stretch the hip flexors and upper thigh (quadriceps). After holding for 45 to 60 seconds, bring the hands to the hips and the torso more upright to increase the stretch (2). Hold again for 45 to 60 seconds. Change sides. Be sure to keep the pelvis level with both hip bones square to the front of your mat. Inner unit on!

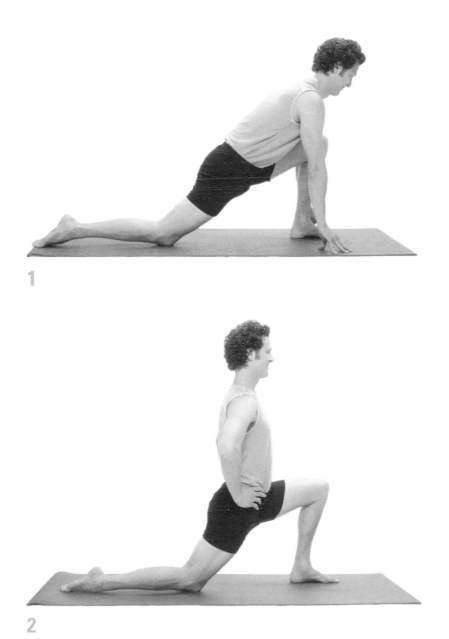

Pelvic Peel and Hinge

Begin lying on your back with the feet flat on the floor, knees bent, heels in line with the sit bones, and arms next to your trunk with the palms down (1). Place a rolled towel or small ball between the inner thighs. For both variations, use your inner thighs to draw the tailbone away from you when rolling down to feel a tractioning length through the spine. Be sure to coordinate breath with movement.

Peel: Inhale. As you exhale, slowly peel the spine away from the floor starting at the tailbone (2), and articulate through each vertebra until your hips are in a straight, diagonal line with the shoulders and knees (3). Inhale again. As you exhale, begin returning to the starting position from the upper back, articulating through each vertebra using the abdominals. Focus on spinal *articulation* in upward and downward movement.

Hinge: Inhale. As you exhale, bring the pelvis up in one movement and in one piece until it is in a straight diagonal line between the shoulders and knees (3). Inhale again. As you exhale, begin returning to the starting position from the upper back, articulating through each vertebra using the abdominals (4). Focus on pelvic and spinal *stability* in upward movement, spinal *articulation* in downward movement.

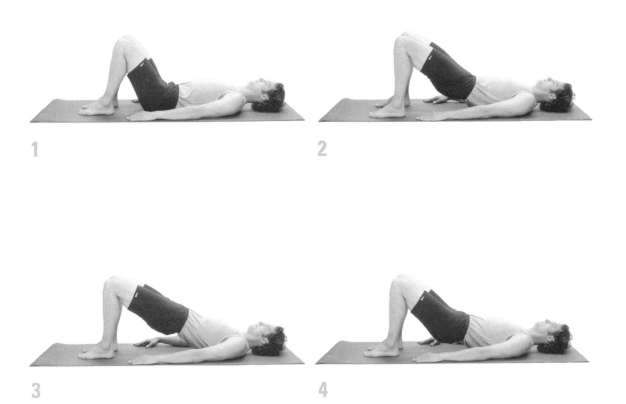

1

2

3

4

Begin lying on your back with the legs parallel and stretched toward the ceiling (1). Softly point the feet. Hold the arms out to the sides in a T position or alongside the torso for greater challenge. If the hamstrings are tight, bend the knees. For added support, you can tie a strength band around the legs above the knees. Keep the pelvis neutral. Inhale as the pelvis tips to one side (2). Exhale as you return the pelvis back to center. Repeat to the other side. As in hip rolls, the upper torso should remain stabilized.

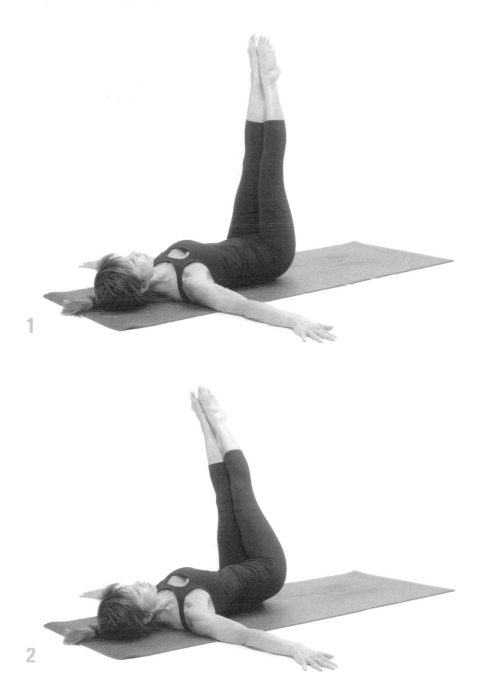

Roll-Down With Strength Band

Begin sitting upright with bent knees and ankles flexed (1). Wrap a strength band around the feet, flat with the top edge of the band covering the toes. Grasp the band near the ankles, and pull it to sit upright. Keep the arms straight at all times! Inhale. As you exhale, slowly roll the spine back beginning with the lower spine as you articulate the vertebrae one at a time to the floor (2) until you are lying down flat (3). Make sure the head arrives last! Keep the arms straight, keep the knees bent, and be mindful not to pull the band with the arms or you will lose the assistance of the band in rolling up and down. Inhale as you curl the head, neck, and shoulders off the floor. Exhale as you continue peeling the spine away from the floor and return to the upright starting position.

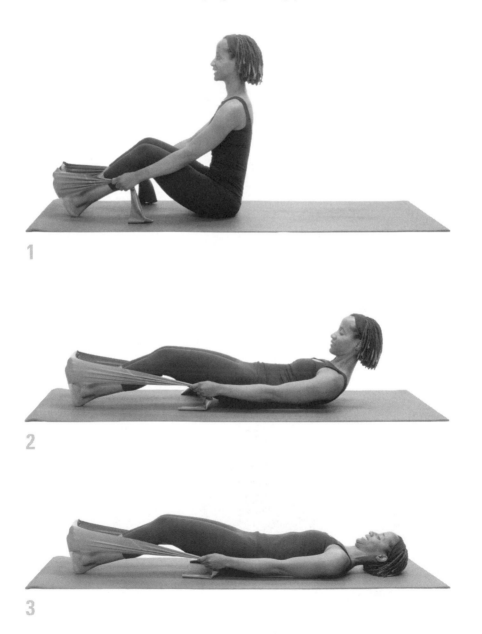

1

2

3

Begin balancing just in front of the tailbone with the knees bent into the chest, head down, and arms wrapped around the outside of the shins (1). Feet are not touching the floor. Abdominal connection and shoulder blade stabilization assist you with your balance. Inhale. As you exhale, roll back (2). Exhale more deeply as you roll back up to balance position (double exhalation). Repeat 6 to 8 breaths. Engage the shoulder blades down the back at all times. Be sure you roll only onto the upper back, never onto your neck. It is important to feel the use of the abdominals as an impetus for the *initiation* of movement as well as to *stop* the movement. Maintain the ball shape throughout the movement phase. You have a choice of handhold positioning: one hand on each ankle, one hand holding the opposite ankle and other hand holding the opposite wrist, or forearms tightly wrapped across shins grasping outside of calves.

This exercise is contraindicated for those participants with thoracic osteoporosis or pre-existing neck issues.

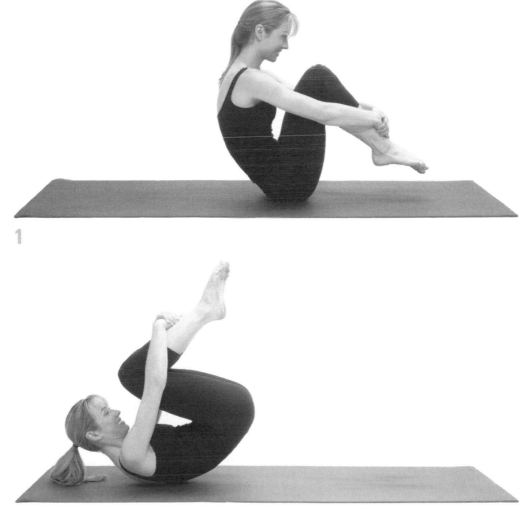

1

2

Rollover

Begin lying on your back with your arms at your sides, palms down, and legs together and reaching to the ceiling with the feet softly pointed (1). If the hamstrings are tight, you may slightly bend the knees. Inhale. As you exhale, begin rolling the pelvis back using the abdominals as you curl the spine (tail end) toward you. Your legs will begin to reach toward your head into a modified plow position (2). Inhale as you open the legs shoulder-distance apart and flex the ankles (3). As you exhale, begin articulating the spine sequentially one vertebra at a time back toward the floor with control (4). Return to the starting position. Inhale as you bring the legs together using the inner thighs, and point the feet. Exhale, and repeat the movements. Repeat 5 times, then repeat 5 more times initiating the rollover with the legs apart. Be sure to "ride the wave of the breath" so that all movements are smooth and controlled. If the hamstrings are tight, be sure to bend the knees slightly.

This exercise is contraindicated for those individuals with thoracic osteoporosis and preexisting neck problems.

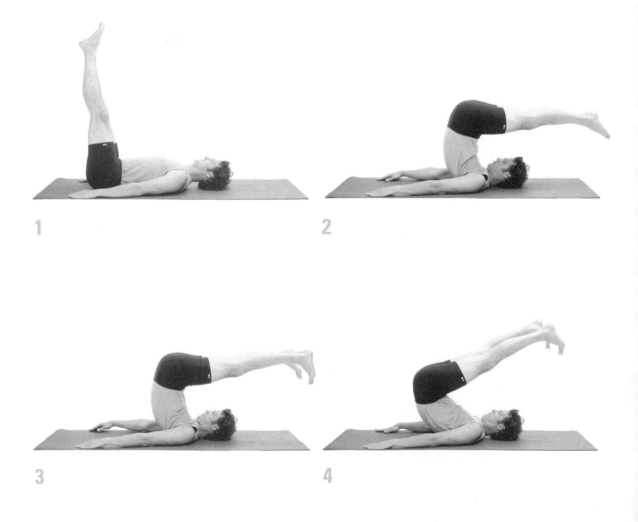

1

2

3

4

Roll-Up With Shoulder Rotation

Begin lying on your back with the arms reaching beside the ears, grasping a strength band (1). The legs are straight and slightly apart with the ankles flexed. Inhale as you bring the arms up perpendicular to the floor, keeping the band taut between the hands (2); and curl the upper torso forward bringing the head in between the arms. Exhaling, lower the arms over the legs and smoothly articulate the spine up using abdominal control until you are reaching the arms long over the legs parallel to the floor (3). Inhale sitting upright (4), and rotate the arms upward and then behind you, stretching open the chest and shoulders and stretching the band if needed (5). Exhale as the arms continue down behind you. Inhale, and bring the arms back up and around to the front, and flex the spine forward, arms once again parallel to the floor (3). Exhale as you articulate the spine one vertebra at a time back down to the starting position. Be sure to keep the shoulder blades anchored on the back as you go through the arm movement and chest stretch.

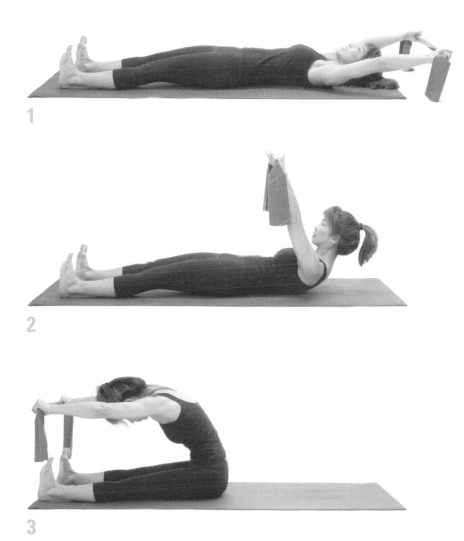

(continued)

Roll-Up With Shoulder Rotation (continued)

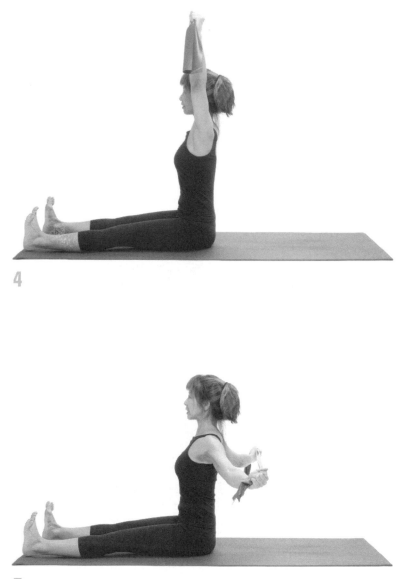

4

5

Seated Abduction and Adduction

Begin seated upright with the legs straight in front of you and apart approximately 90 degrees, the ankles flexed, and the arms open to the sides parallel to the floor, palms facing forward (1). You may place your hands on the floor if necessary (4). Bend both knees slightly if it is difficult to sit upright with a neutral pelvis. Inhale as you lengthen the spine and prepare. As you exhale, bring your left leg across to close and meet the right leg using the inner thigh muscles (2). Inhale as you return that leg open to the starting position. Exhale as you bring the right leg in to meet the left leg (3). Repeat for 5 sets. Feel a tension connection between the inner thighs and multifidus. You may reverse breathing on the movement phase.

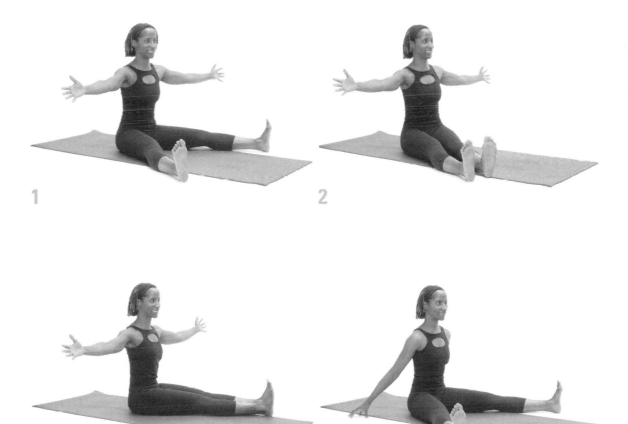

1

2

3

4

Seated Shoulder Stretch

Seated upright, grasp a strength band slightly wider than shoulder-width apart with the arms lowered in front of the torso (1). Maintain some tension between the hands, but do not pull. Arms are straight but not locked. Legs are in any position that is comfortable (usually I bend them to cross-legged position) as long as the pelvis stays neutral. Inhaling, bring the arms up in front of you and keep them straight (2). Exhaling, continue to rotate the arms (shoulders) all the way around behind you, feeling a strong stretch in the front of the chest near the shoulders (3). Keep the shoulder blades down! Inhale as you bring the arms up from behind you to above the head again (2). Exhale as you bring the arms back down the front of the torso to the starting position (1). Head and neck should not have to shift for the arms to complete the circle. If you experience strain in the shoulders or neck area, widen the grip between the hands.

Seated Spinal Extension With Arm Support

Sit upright with the legs crossed, hands placed slightly behind the hips on the floor (1). Inhaling, lift the breastbone up toward the ceiling, allowing the entire spine to arch up and back. Exhaling, maximize this position and lean back slightly onto the hands (2). Inhale again in the extended position. When extending the spine, work to distribute the arc evenly from tailbone to crown of head. Strongly engage the deep abdominals and funnel the ribs. Be sure the head is not hanging at the neck. Reach the sternum upward to expand the chest. Breathe deeply for 5 breaths. Exhale, and return the torso upright to the starting position.

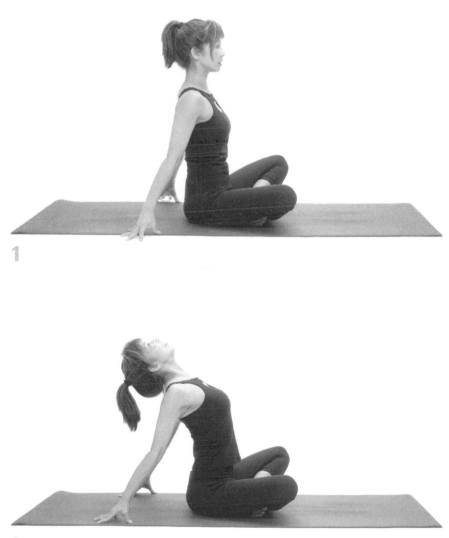

Shoulder Bridge Hold

Begin lying on your back with the knees bent, feet flat, and heels in line with your sitting bones. Place the arms palms down near your hips. Inhale to prepare. As you exhale, bring the hips up in the air beyond diagonal neutral. Roll the shoulders slightly underneath you to reach the breastbone toward your chin. Avoid compressing the chin to the chest. Firmly press the arms into the floor to assist you in spinal extension. Hold this position, and breathe for 6 to 8 breaths. Engage the inner unit. This exercise is a contraction of the back body and an opening and lengthening of the front body. The knees and thighs have a tendency to flare apart, so be sure to press down through the balls of the big toes to engage the inner thighs. On your last exhalation, slowly roll the shoulders out from underneath you and articulate the spine back down to the starting position.

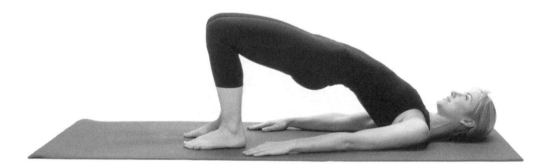

Side Kick

Begin lying on your side, the bottom leg with knee bent behind you, thighs parallel. Reach the bottom arm over head and place your head on a small pillow on the arm. Place the top arm in front of your chest to assist with balance. Keep the entire torso in a straight line. The top leg is straight with the toes pointed (1). Inhale as you bring the top leg to parallel to the floor, reaching long out of the hips. Exhale as you maintain this position with the deep abdominals and back muscles. Inhale again, and bring the top leg forward, flexing at the hip and ankle (2). Exhale, point the foot, and carry the leg back behind you, only as far as you can maintain your stabilized torso (3). Be sure to feel leg movement, not pelvic movement.

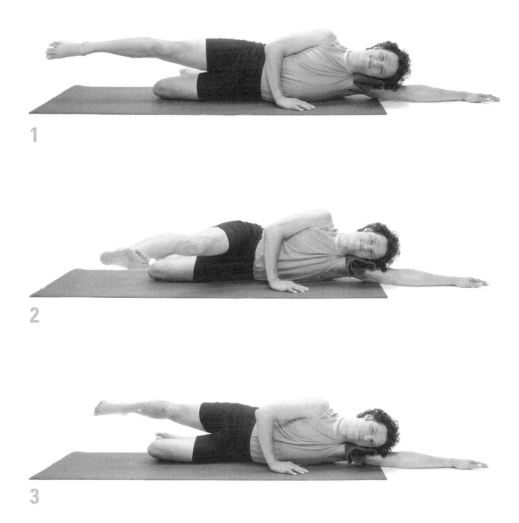

1

2

3

Single-Leg Kick

Begin lying on the floor belly down, propped up on your elbows with the hands made into fists (1). Place the elbows directly below the shoulders, and keep the forearms angled in so that the fists are together. Extend the legs straight behind you very close together. Strongly engage the inner unit, and keep the pubic bone anchored on the mat. As you inhale, bend the knee with the ankle flexed and pulse twice gently toward the buttock (2). As you exhale, slowly extend the leg and return it to the starting position (3). Repeat with the other leg. Be sure to resist the movement of straightening the knee with your hamstrings. You may place your head down on your hands if the lower back feels compressed.

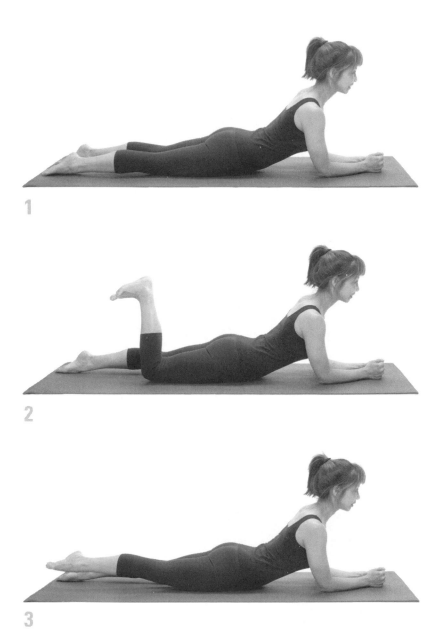

1

2

3

Single-Leg Stretch

Begin lying on your back with the pelvis in neutral. Bring one knee toward the chest with the outside hand placed at the ankle and the inside hand placed at the same knee (1). Reach the other leg long into the distance, bringing it to about a 45-degree angle or lower if you have no back strain. Inhale as you switch legs, changing hand position as well (2). Exhale as you switch leg and hand position again. Be sure to keep the elbows wide with the shoulders down. It is hand over hand to change hand position with the leg switch.

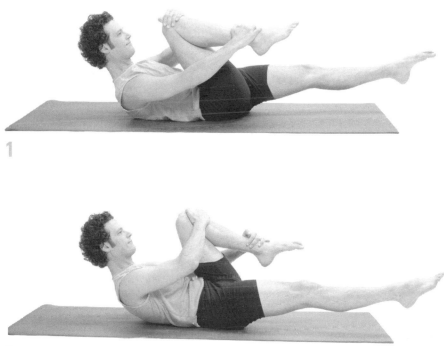

Slow Arrow

Lying on your belly, reach the arms long next to the torso, palms facing inward, legs parallel, approximately 4 inches (10 centimeters) apart (1). Place a small towel or pillow under the forehead. Inhale to prepare. As you exhale, hover the chest off of the floor, head and neck following (2). Reach the arms toward the feet off of the floor and next to the trunk. Inhale. As you exhale, bring the arms around to form the letter T (3) and continue toward the head, with the arms rotating to form a V shape (4). Inhale. As you exhale, return the arms in a semicircle back to the starting position and lower the trunk and head back down. Legs remain on the floor at all times. Be sure to engage the inner unit and feel the arm movement coordinated with the breath. As the arms are moving in the semicircle shape, the shoulder blades must remain anchored down on the back.

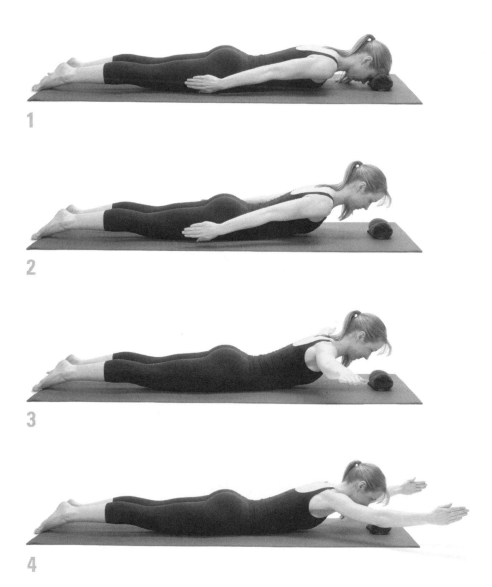

Slow Swim

Begin lying on your belly with the arms reaching forward alongside the ears and the legs parallel and stretching out behind you in line with your sit bones. Hover the face off of the floor while aligning the head and neck with the rest of the spine. Inhale. As you exhale, float the opposite arm and leg slightly off the floor, reaching them long (1). Inhale as you return them back to the floor. Exhale and reach the opposing leg and arm (2), and inhale returning them back to the floor. Be sure not to disturb the levelness of your pelvis and shoulder girdle. To challenge respiratory strength, you may try two movements per inhalation and two movements per exhalation.

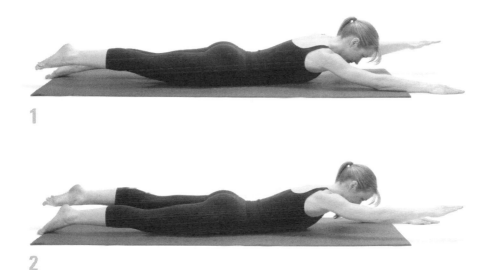

Spine Spiral With Arms Crossed

Begin seated upright with the legs crossed at the ankles and the knees bent and open (1). Position the arms at shoulder height, elbows bent with the forearms stacked on top of one another. Inhaling, rotate the upper torso in one direction (2). As you exhale, begin to rotate the torso back to starting position. Initiate your rotation from the lower ribs and keep your arms low in front of your chest. Imagine you are spiraling upward. Repeat the movement to the other side.

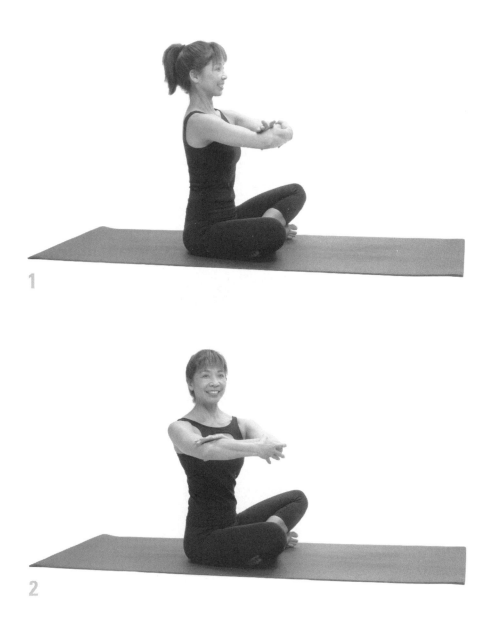

Spine Spiral With Elbow Extension

Begin seated upright with the legs crossed at the ankles and the knees bent and open (1). Place the arms in front of your chest, bent at the elbows with fingertips touching. Inhaling, begin to rotate the upper torso to the right, extending the right elbow in that direction (2). As you exhale, begin to rotate the torso back to the starting position, folding the elbow back in. Begin your rotation from the lower ribs, and use the extension of the elbow to assist in deepening the rotation. Keep the arms low across the chest to avoid elevating the shoulders. Imagine you are spiraling upward to keep the length in the spine. Repeat the movement to the other side.

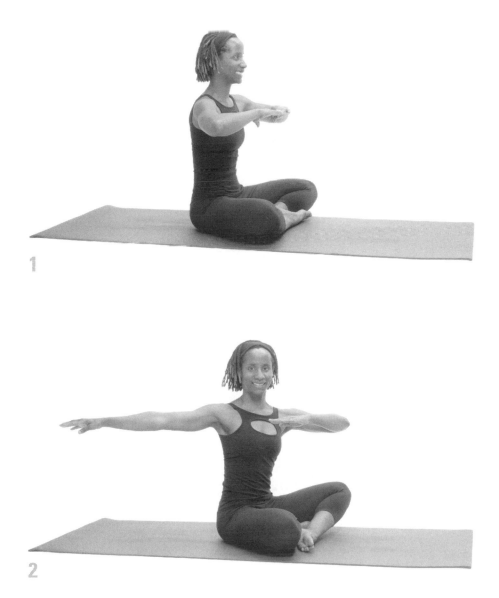

1

2

Spine Stretch

Begin sitting upright with the legs stretched in front of you straight and opened to approximately 90 degrees with the ankles flexed (1). Bend the knees if hamstring shortness prevents an upright neutral pelvis. Stretch the arms in front of you, parallel to the floor, at shoulder height with the palms down. Inhale to prepare and lengthen the spine. As you exhale, flex the spine forward until the fingertips touch the floor (2). Inhale in this position. Exhaling, slide the fingers forward, increasing the flexion of the spine. Avoid collapsing in the chest, and do not elevate the shoulders. Inhale in the flexed spine position. As you exhale, return the spine, vertebra by vertebra, to the upright starting position.

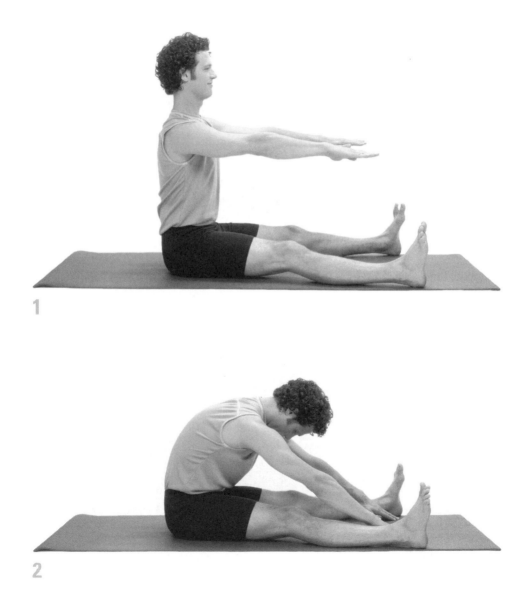

1

2

Swan

Begin lying facedown with the hands placed flat near the shoulders and the elbows bent and pointing toward the legs (1). Reach the legs behind you, straight, slightly turned out, approximately 6 to 8 inches (15 to 20 centimeters) apart. Inhale. As you exhale, slowly arc the upper trunk away from the floor using the back muscles (2). Press lightly into the hands to assist you in your spinal extension. Inhale as you lower the torso back down. As you exhale, reach the legs long into a distance and hover them slightly above the floor (3). Inhale, returning the legs to the floor. Exhale, and repeat the upper trunk and leg movements. Be sure to feel leg movement, not pelvic movement. Repeat 6 sets (upper- and lower-body movements).

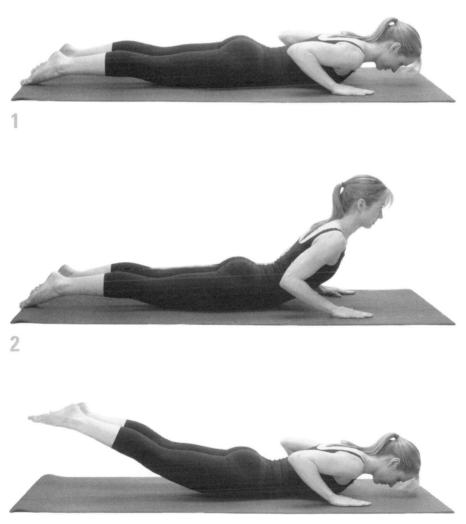

1

2

3

5

Moderate
Workouts

20-Minute Moderate Workout

The 20-minute moderate workout provides a quick, concise, middle-of-the-road morning challenge for those of you who are comfortable with the Pilates method. When you are sufficiently experienced in working at a moderate pace and intensity, flowing from one exercise to the next gives you the added benefit of physical and mental endurance. If you have a little more than 20 minutes but less than 40, squeeze in a few extra repetitions here and there (especially the exercises that may not be your favorites), and you will feel very satisfied with yourself when you finish!

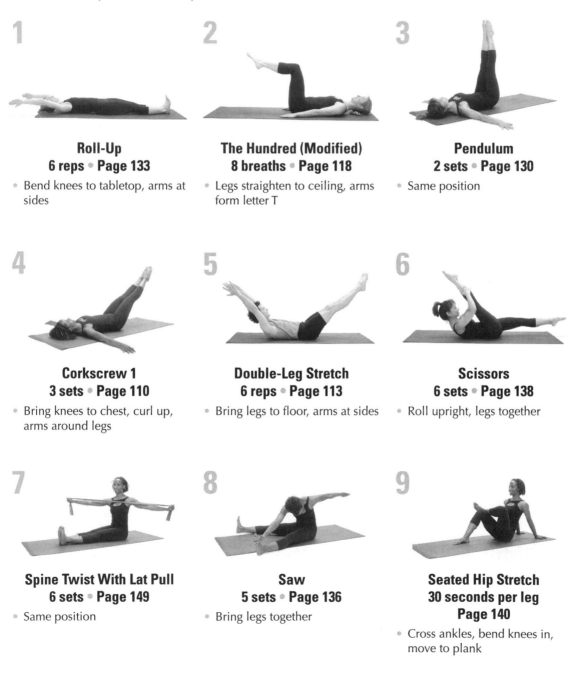

1
Roll-Up
6 reps • Page 133
- Bend knees to tabletop, arms at sides

2
The Hundred (Modified)
8 breaths • Page 118
- Legs straighten to ceiling, arms form letter T

3
Pendulum
2 sets • Page 130
- Same position

4
Corkscrew 1
3 sets • Page 110
- Bring knees to chest, curl up, arms around legs

5
Double-Leg Stretch
6 reps • Page 113
- Bring legs to floor, arms at sides

6
Scissors
6 sets • Page 138
- Roll upright, legs together

7
Spine Twist With Lat Pull
6 sets • Page 149
- Same position

8
Saw
5 sets • Page 136
- Bring legs together

9
Seated Hip Stretch
30 seconds per leg
Page 140
- Cross ankles, bend knees in, move to plank

10

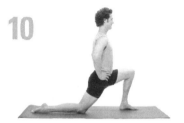

Lunge With Hands at Hips
30 to 60 seconds per leg
Page 123

- Step leg back to plank

11

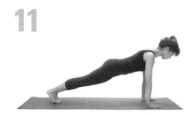

Front Support
6 sets
(Push-ups are optional)
Page 116

- Hinge back into downward dog

12

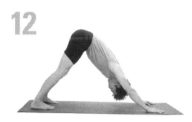

Downward Dog
5 long breaths • Page 114

- Hinge to plank, lower body to floor

13

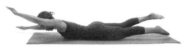

Swimming
6 breaths • Page 151

- Sweep arms around behind back, turn head

14

Double-Leg Kick
6 sets • Page 112

- Turn to lie on one side

15

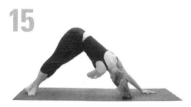

Twist
5 times per side • Page 152

- Turn to sit upright

16

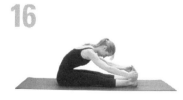

Forward Bend
5 to 10 breaths • Page 115

- Roll down to lie on back

17

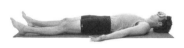

Corpse
3 to 5 minutes • Page 111

40-Minute Moderate Workout

The 40-minute moderate workout is geared for those days when you are not as crunched for time but still cannot waste any moments either. Designed for those of you who have a solid foundation of strength and understanding of the Pilates approach, this workout will thoroughly give you the upper-body strengthening, spinal articulation for fluidity, and deep-back and abdominal strengthening that Pilates is famous for, all while challenging your ability to keep the flow.

1

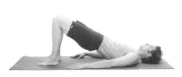

Pelvic Peel • Page 129
- Alternate with ab curl for 6 sets

2

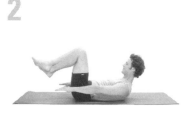

Ab Curl • Page 103
- Bring legs to tabletop, arms at sides

3

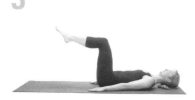

**The Hundred
8 breaths • Page 117**
- Straighten legs to ceiling

4

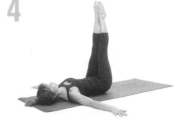

**Pendulum
3 sets • Page 130**
- Same position

5

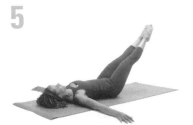

**Corkscrew 1
5 sets • Page 110**
- Lower legs to floor

6

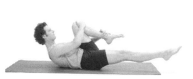

**Single-Leg Stretch
6 sets • Page 145**
- Same position

7

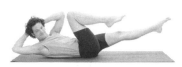

**Oblique Rotation
6 sets • Page 127**
- Roll up to seated, open legs

8

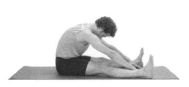

**Spine Stretch With Extension
6 sets • Page 147**
- Bring legs together, grasp band

9

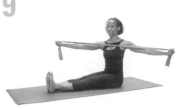

**Spine Twist With Lat Pull
8 sets • Page 149**
- Bend knees to chest, wrap arms around legs

10

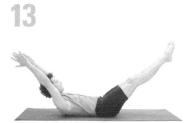

Rolling
6 sets • Page 131

- Stretch legs forward, hands behind on floor

11

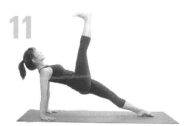

Back Support
(With Leg Raise)
4 sets • Page 105

- Sit up, open legs, arms to I position

12

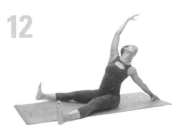

Saw With Back Extension
5 sets • Page 137

- Roll down to lying on back

13

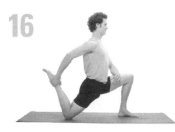

Double-Leg Stretch
8 sets • Page 113

- Bring both legs to floor, arms to T position

14

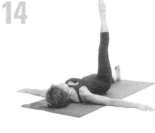

Leg Circles
5 sets each direction
Page 122

- Roll up, cross ankles, bend knees, plank

15

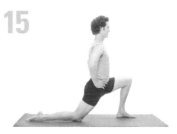

Lunge With Hands at Hips
30 to 60 seconds per side
Page 123

- Same position

16

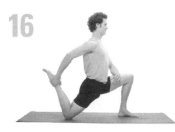

Lunge With Quadriceps
Stretch
30 to 60 seconds per side
Page 124

- Move into plank

17

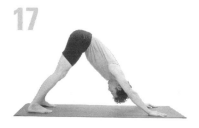

Downward Dog
5 long breaths • Page 114

- Lower torso to floor

18

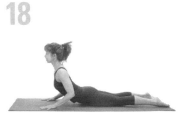

Swan (Modified Rocking)
6 to 8 reps • Page 150

- Reach arms around to grasp ankles

(continued)

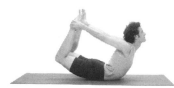

19

Bow (Holding)
3 to 4 sets • Page 106

- Release ankles, press up to plank

20

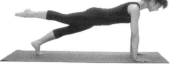

Front Support With Push-Ups
6 sets • Page 116

- Lower torso to floor

21

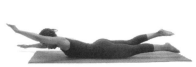

Swimming
6 breaths • Page 151

- Turn to one side

22

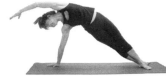

Side Kick, Propped on Elbow
6 sets per side • Page 144

- Same position

23

Side Bend
6 sets • Page 143

- Turn over to lie on back

24

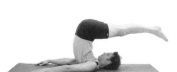

Rollover
4 sets • Page 132

- Same position

25

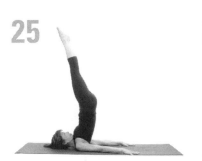

Jackknife
5 sets • Page 119

- Bend knees, feet flat, arms at sides

26

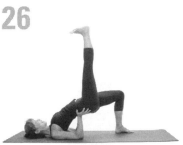

Shoulder Bridge With
Leg Pulse
3 sets per leg • Page 142

- Lower hips, stretch arms and legs out

27

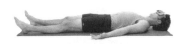

Corpse
Maintain for minimum of
3 minutes • Page 111

Finally, you have a full hour to focus on gleaning all the benefits that Pilates is famous for. Included in this workout are the classic versions of both the swan and the bow, both rocking, as well as a couple of smooth, creative transitions from one exercise to the next (arrow double salute into swimming and side bend into front support into side bend). Keep your attention focused on the quality of your movements, and perhaps put some extra emphasis on your breath control, which is always an excellent choice for sustaining your mental edge.

1

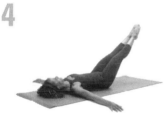

Roll-Up With Strength Band and Shoulder Rotation
8 sets • Page 134

- Bend knees to tabletop, arms at sides

2

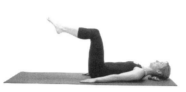

The Hundred
8 breaths • Page 117

- Straighten legs to ceiling

3

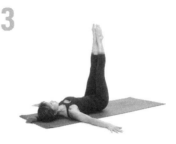

Pendulum
3 sets • Page 130

- Same position

4

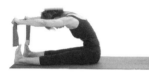

Corkscrew 1
8 sets • Page 110

- Lower legs to floor, roll up

5

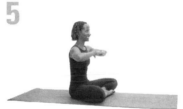

Spine Spiral With Double Pulse
8 sets • Page 146

- Bend knees to chest, wrap arms around legs

6

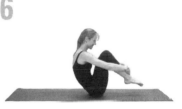

Rolling
8 sets • Page 131

- Roll back to floor

7

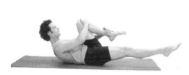

Single-Leg Stretch
8 sets (inhale for 2 changes)
Page 145

- Straighten bent leg to ceiling

8

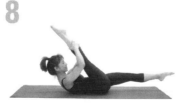

Scissors
8 sets • Page 138

- Fold knees to chest, wrap arms, torso up

9

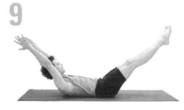

Double-Leg Stretch
8 sets • Page 113

- Legs to floor, lie down on back

(continued)

10

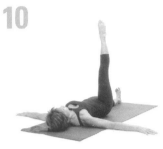

Leg Circles
**5 times each direction
per leg • Page 122**
- Roll up to seated

11

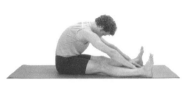

Spine Stretch With Extension
6 sets • Page 147
- Same position

12

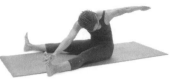

Saw
6 sets • Page 136
- Roll down to lying on back

13

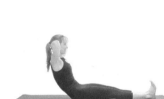

Neck Pull
5 sets • Page 125
- Roll up, grasp band

14

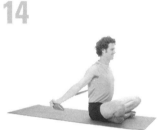

Seated Shoulder Stretch
5 sets • Page 141
- Moving to a kneeling position

15

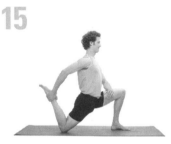

**Lunge With
Quadriceps Stretch**
1 minute per side • Page 124
- Back leg forward, sit, stretch
  legs to front

16

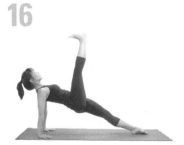

**Back Support
(With Leg Raise)**
6 sets • Page 105
- Bend knees in and open

17

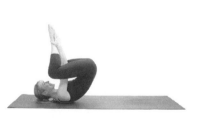

Seal
6 sets • Page 139
- Bring legs to open V position,
  grasp ankles

18

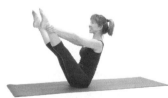

Open-Leg Rocker
6 sets • Page 128
- Bring legs together (remain up),
  torso rolls down

19

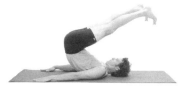

Rollover
4 sets per direction
Page 132

- Turn over onto front, arms at sides

20

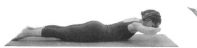

Arrow With Double Salute
5 sets • Page 104

- Sweep arms around to reach overhead

21

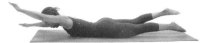

Swimming
8 breaths • Page 151

- Roll onto side

22

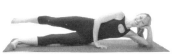

Side Kick, Propped on Elbow
6 sets per side • Page 144

- Same position

23

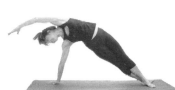

Side Bend (One Side)
5 sets • Page 143

- Turn facedown to plank

24

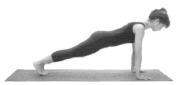

Front Support With Push-Ups
5 sets • Page 116

- Turn to one side

25

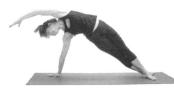

Side Bend (Other Side)
5 sets • Page 143

- Turn to face floor, knees down

26

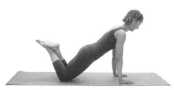

Knee Push-Up
8 sets • Page 121

- Lower torso to floor, straighten legs

27

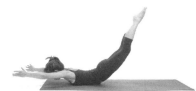

Swan (Modified Rocking)
8 to 10 sets • Page 150

- Come up to hands and knees

(continued)

28

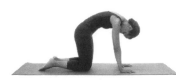

Cat Stretch
4 sets • Page 108
- Lower torso to floor

29

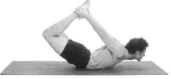

Bow (Rocking)
6 to 8 breaths • Page 107
- Come up to hands and knees

30

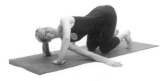

Cat Twist
4 sets • Page 109
- Turn over to lie on back

31

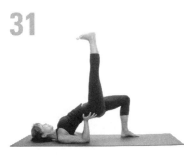

Shoulder Bridge With
Leg Pulse
5 sets • Page 142
- Bend knees to chest, cross legs at knee

32

Knee Over Knee
Twist Stretch
30 to 60 seconds per side
Page 120

Ab Curl

Begin lying on your back, place your feet flat on the floor (1) or legs in the air with knees bent at 90-degree angles, ankles crossed, knees open above the hips. Bend the knees, and align the heels with the sit bones. Place the arms next to your trunk with the palms down. Put a small ball or rolled towel between the inner thighs. Inhale. As you exhale, bring the upper torso forward, hinging at the T point (located straight back to the spine from the lowest point of the breastbone), arms reaching toward the feet and hovering parallel to the floor (2). Breathe in for 3 counts, and breathe out for 4 counts for 6 complete cycles. Inhale for a seventh breath. As you exhale, slowly return the torso back to the starting position using the abdominals. Maintain a neutral pelvis during the entire exercise.

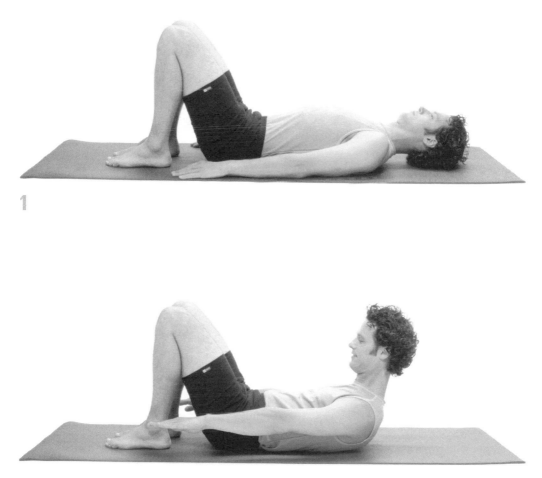

1

2

Arrow With Double Salute

Begin facedown with your head turned to the right (1). Arms are alongside the torso with the palms up. Legs stretch back with the heels in line with the sit bones. Inhaling, hover the torso while simultaneously bringing both hands toward the forehead, fingers lightly touching the forehead in a double salute (2). Bend the elbows, and turn the face toward the floor. Exhale as you return arms and torso to the starting position, turning the head to the left as you come to the floor. Be sure to anchor the pelvis by engaging the inner unit, and keep your shoulder blades stabilized. Legs may hover as well to increase challenge.

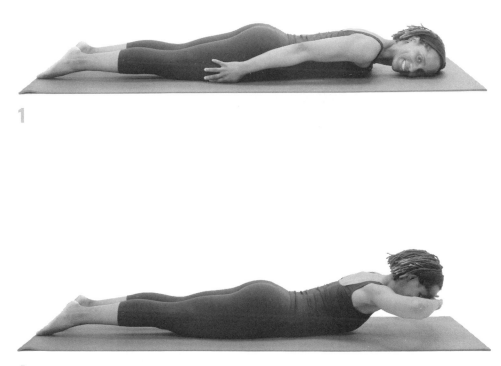

1

2

Back Support

From a seated position with the legs together and the hands placed behind the hips, lift your pelvis until it is in one straight line between the shoulders and feet (1). Keep the head and neck in line with the rest of the spine. Inhaling, bring the right leg straight up with a flexed ankle and pulse gently twice (2). Distribute the workload throughout the entire body so that you don't overly fatigue the arms and shoulders. Press the soles of the feet into the floor as much as possible. If the calves cramp from lack of ankle flexibility, keep the heels in strong contact with the floor to engage the entire back of the legs. Press the inner thighs firmly together, and avoid allowing the legs to roll apart. Exhaling, return the right leg back to the starting position. Inhaling, bring the left leg up with the ankle flexed and pulse gently twice. Exhaling, return the left leg back to the starting position.

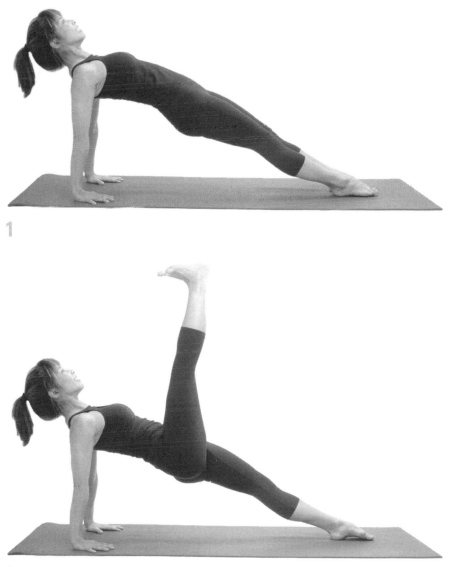

1

2

Bow (Holding)

Lying facedown, bend both knees, and grasp the ankles (1). If possible, keep the feet touching. Inhaling, engage the inner unit. Exhaling, simultaneously press the ankles against the hands and bring the upper trunk into extension (2). The thighs may or may not touch the floor. Holding this bow position, breathe deeply for 5 to 6 complete breaths, then return back to the starting position on the last exhalation. When breathing and holding bow pose, be sure to bring yourself just to approximately 75 percent of your maximally stretched position and relax there so that the breath can be long and steady. If the breath becomes strained or ragged, you have pushed beyond the ability of your body to maintain the position with ease.

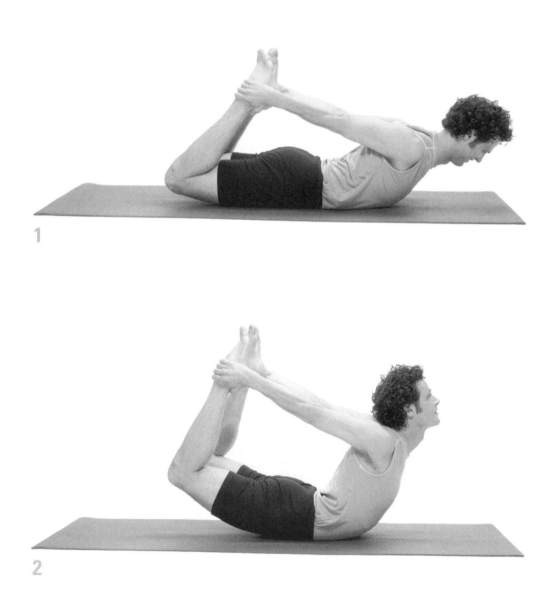

1

2

Bow (Rocking)

Lying facedown, bend both knees, and grasp the ankles (1). If possible, keep the feet touching. Inhaling, engage the inner unit. Exhaling, simultaneously press the ankles against the hands and bring the upper trunk into extension. The thighs may or may not touch the floor. Inhaling, gently rock the upper torso up with the chest lifted (2). Exhaling, gently rock the upper torso forward onto the chest, keeping the head lifted (3). Be aware not to initiate the rocking movement by jerking the head up and down. This extremely demanding position requires flexibility at the hip flexors, shoulder joints, quadriceps, and spine.

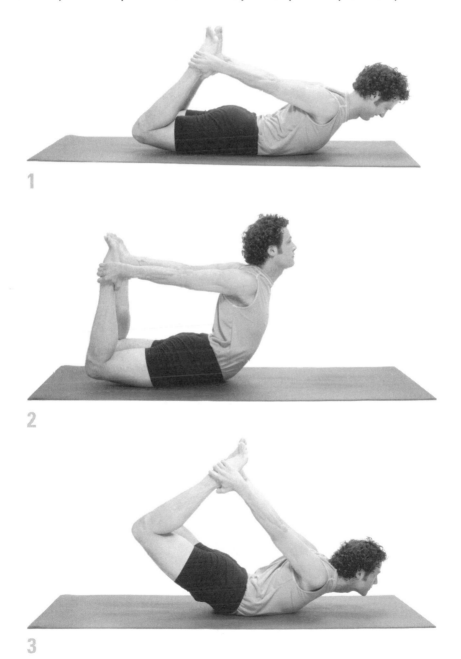

1

2

3

Cat Stretch

Begin in a quadruped position with the hands directly beneath the shoulders and the knees directly below the hips (1). Maintain a neutral pelvis and stabilized shoulder girdle. Align the head and neck with the rest of the spine. Inhale. As you exhale, begin to contract the deep abdominals and gently curve the spine into a convex arch so that the spine is flexed and curved toward the ceiling (2). Inhale. As you exhale, begin to articulate through the spinal column as you move from the flexed position to an extended, arched position (3). Avoid hunching the shoulders by using the scapulae stabilizers to draw the shoulder blades down the back whether in a flexed or extended spinal position. Allow the breath to carry the movement like a wave rippling through the spine. Avoid overworking. This movement is meant to alleviate any accumulated tension in the body. Repeat 4 or 5 sets.

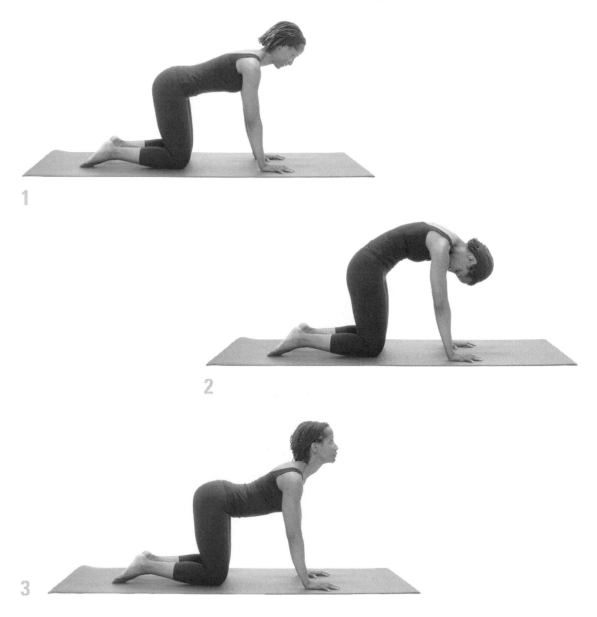

Cat Twist

Begin in a quadruped position with the hands directly beneath the shoulders and knees directly beneath the hips. As you inhale, turn the left arm inward, pointing the fingers toward the chest with the elbow jutting outward and slightly upward. As you exhale, reach the right arm under the left, rotating the torso (spine) to look over the top of your left shoulder (1). Allow the spine to rotate and fully arch from tailbone to head at the same time, pulling the chest through. Avoid overturning the neck and keep the chin aligned with the breastbone. Do not look underneath the top arm. Repeat to the opposite side (2).

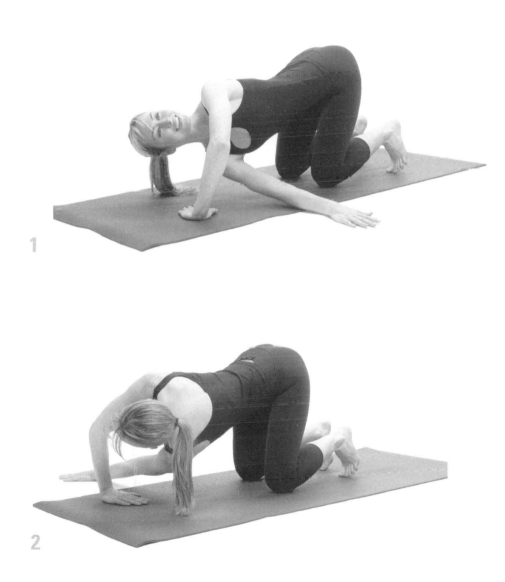

Corkscrew 1

Begin lying on your back with legs up toward ceiling, parallel and pressed together, feet softly pointed (1). Place your arms to form a letter T, or for a greater challenge, place them alongside the torso. Bend the knees if hamstring tightness does not allow you to keep your pelvis neutral. Inhaling, tilt the pelvis to one side (2). Exhaling, rotate the pelvis away from you (3, lower spine is slightly arching) around to the opposite side (4), then back to center starting position. Inhaling, tip the pelvis to the other side. Exhaling, rotate the pelvis away from you, around to the other side, and back to starting position. The upper torso should remain stabilized, and the opposing back rib cage should not leave the floor. Continue to alternate sides.

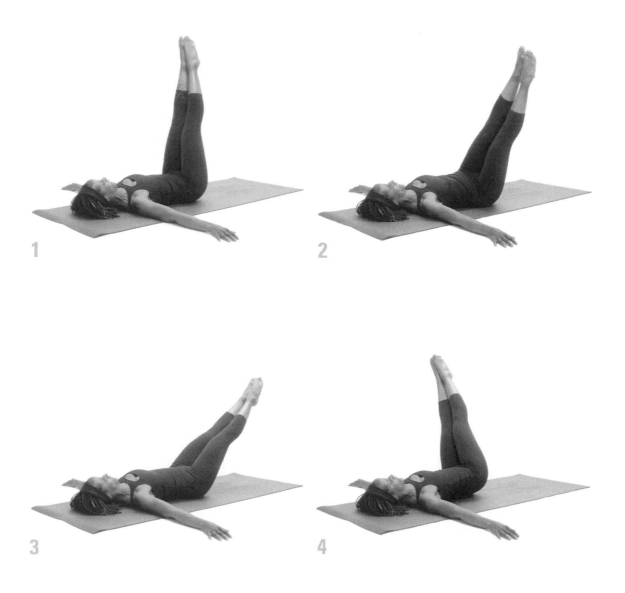

Corpse

Begin lying on your back with the arms out and away from the torso and the palms up. Position the legs slightly apart, and let them flop open. Close your eyes and mouth, and relax your jaw. With each progressive breath, allow your face to soften, the corners of your mouth to release, and the space between your eyebrows to open. Feel the tension drain from your body like grains of sands dribbling through an hourglass, slowly and steadily with each subsequent breath. Breathe deeply and completely. Let go.

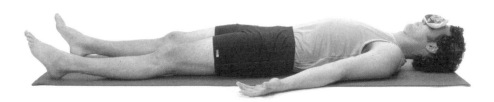

Double-Leg Kick

Lie facedown with the legs together, arms behind you, elbows bent and resting on floor, with your hands at your lower back (1). Head is turned to one side. Engage the inner unit. As you inhale, bend the knees and pulse the heels toward the buttocks 3 times (2). As you exhale, stretch the arms out behind you with the palms facing inward, stretch the legs long and reach them slightly off the floor, and arch the entire upper torso (3). Keep head and neck in line with the rest of your spine. Inhaling, return to the starting position with your head now turned to the other side. Be sure that the elbows relax toward the floor before you repeat the next sequence.

Note: Elbows may or may not be completely resting on the floor. *Do not force elbows to the floor.*

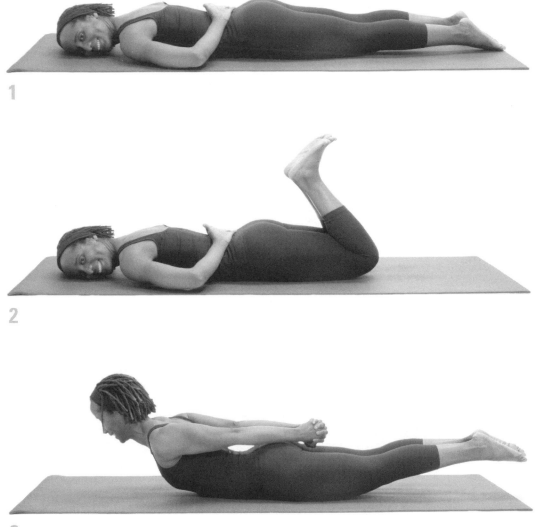

Double-Leg Stretch

Begin lying on your back, knees bent toward the chest, legs together, and feet softly pointed (1). Upper torso is curled forward with the arms reaching toward the ankles on the outside of the legs. Pelvis is in neutral. As you inhale, reach the arms toward the ceiling and back until they are alongside the ears (2). Simultaneously straighten the legs forward about 45 degrees. As you exhale, sweep the arms to the side (3) and forward while bending the knees back to the starting position. Avoid moving the trunk and especially the head and neck when sweeping the arms. Keep the eyes focused forward and *do not* allow the gaze of the eyes to travel upward, or the head will fall back and strain the neck.

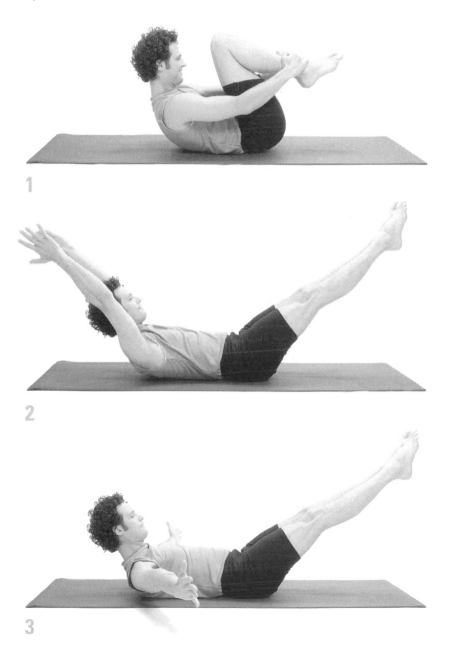

1

2

3

Downward Dog

From a plank position, separate the legs hip-distance apart and press the hips back and up in the air so that the arms, spine, and pelvis form one long diagonal. Press the heels down toward the floor, and fully engage the legs on all sides. Distribute the weight as much as possible onto the legs. Arms are shoulder-distance apart with the neck long. Engage the shoulder blade stabilizers, and lengthen between the armpit and upper side ribs. Be sure that you press the roots of the fingers (located on the palm side of the hand where the large finger knuckles are located) into the floor to avoid bearing all your weight on the base of the palms. Do not allow the ribs to sag toward the floor. The head and neck are in alignment with the rest of the spine. This is a transitional position between exercises. You may also opt to simply rest in child's pose for a less challenging option.

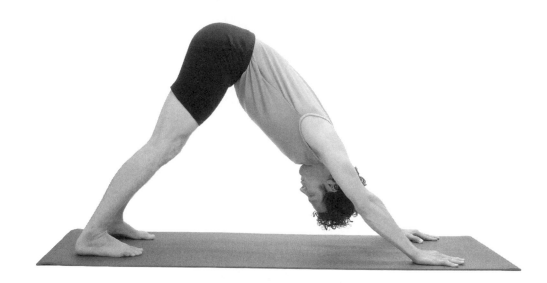

Forward Bend

Begin seated with both legs straight out in front of you together with the ankles flexed. Bend the knees slightly if the hamstrings feel extremely tight. Inhaling, reach the arms up toward the ceiling alongside the ears, palms facing in (1). Exhaling, begin to flex the torso forward over the legs, reaching the hands toward the feet (2). Stay in this position for 5 to 10 deep breaths. You may put a large pillow between your chest and thighs so that the torso may rest on it with the head turned to one side. Be sure to keep the abdominals engaged as well as the legs. If your hands reach your feet, grasp them on the outside to assist in drawing the torso forward. If not, use a strap around the feet to assist in the folding forward.

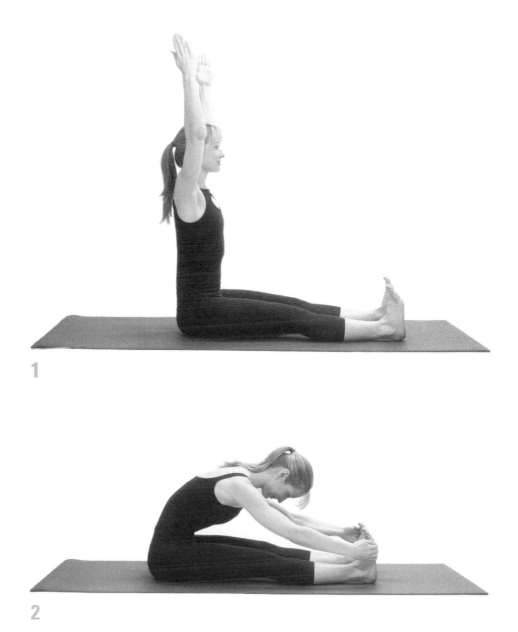

1

2

Front Support With Push-Ups

From a quadruped position, bring the feet back with the legs pressed together so that you form a plank shape (1). Hips are in one straight line between your head and neck, shoulders, and knees. Engage the scapulae stabilizers along with the inner unit and lower glutes. Inhale. As you exhale, pulse the leg up behind you twice only as far up that you do not disturb the stability of the pelvis, spine, and shoulders (2). Inhaling, lower the leg. Repeat with the other leg. Feel a tension connection from the inner thighs through the pelvic floor to the deep abdominals. Watch that the head and neck do not drop. (I call this "falling into the feedbag.") Add push-ups (3) in at either of these points: between each leg pulse (i.e., pulse right leg twice, perform 1 to 3 push-ups, pulse left leg twice, perform 1 to 3 push-ups) or between sets of leg pulses (i.e., pulse right leg twice, then left leg twice, and perform 1 to 3 push-ups; repeat). All push-ups can be done from the knees-on-floor position.

1

2

3

The Hundred

Begin lying on your back, with the legs in the air and pressed strongly together (1). Hips and knees are bent at 90-degree angles, and shins are parallel to the floor. Legs are in a tabletop position (more challenging) or crossed at the ankles with the knees apart (less challenging). Arms are next to your trunk with the palms down. Inhale. As you exhale, bring the upper torso forward, hinging at the T point (located straight back to the spine from the lowest point of the breastbone), and extend the legs straight out about 45 degrees, feet pointed, legs turned out slightly (2). Pumping the arms up and down, inhale for 5 counts, and exhale for 5 counts. Perform 8 complete cycles. Inhale once again, and as you exhale, slowly return the torso and legs back to the starting position using the abdominals. Be sure to keep the pelvis in neutral and the distance from lower rib to hip bones long. Lengthen across the collarbones as you keep the shoulder blades moving down the back. Keep your eyes focused forward toward the inner thighs.

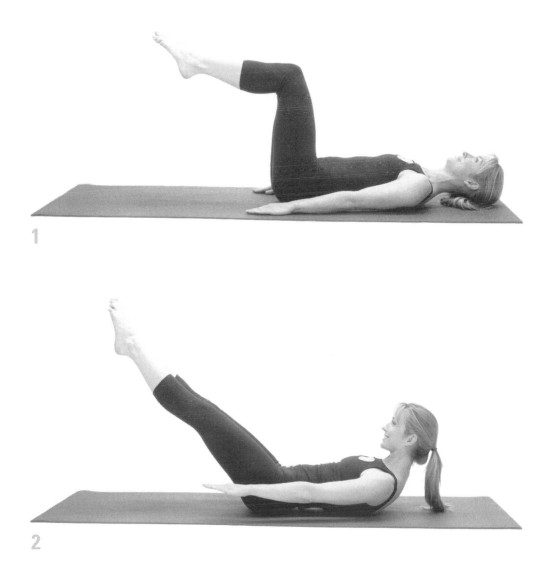

1

2

The Hundred (Modified)

Begin lying on your back, with the legs in the air and pressed strongly together. Hips and knees are bent at 90-degree angles, and shins are parallel to the floor (1). Legs are in a tabletop position (more challenging) or crossed at the ankles with the knees apart (less challenging). Arms are next to your trunk with the palms down. Inhale. As you exhale, bring the upper torso forward, hinging at the T point (located straight back to the spine from the lowest point of the breastbone), with the arms reaching toward the feet, hovering parallel to the floor (2). Pumping the arms up and down, inhale for 5 counts, and exhale for 5 counts. Perform 8 complete cycles. Inhale once again, and as you exhale, engage the abdominals to slowly return the torso back to the starting position. Be sure to keep the pelvis in neutral and the distance from the lower rib to hip bones long. Lengthen across the collar bones as you keep the shoulder blades moving down the back. Keep your eyes focused forward toward the inner thighs.

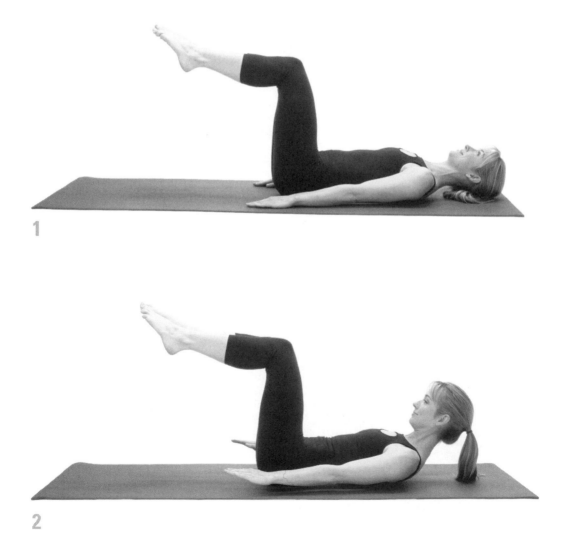

1

2

Jackknife

Lying on your back with the legs together, reach the legs straight up for the ceiling, forming a 90-degree angle at the hip joint (1). If your hamstrings are restricting this position, slightly bend the knees. Strongly use the inner thigh muscles to keep the legs together throughout this exercise. Arms are alongside the torso, palms facing down. Inhaling, deeply engage the abdominals to tilt the pelvis back. Do not initiate movement from the legs; they are just along for the ride. Exhaling, engage the hamstrings and glutes to reach the legs overhead to a plow position (2) and then straight up to a shoulder stand (3). Strongly recruit the leg muscles to achieve this position. Inhaling, fold at the hip joint back to about 45 degrees (4). Exhaling, control the articulation of the spine back down to the starting position while reaching the legs strongly in the opposite direction. Avoid dropping the legs toward the chest, and keep the hip joint open.

This exercise is contraindicated for those with neck issues as well as those with thoracic osteoporosis.

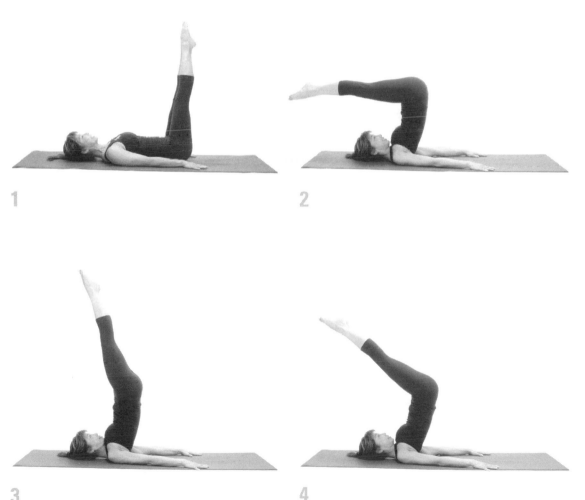

1

2

3

4

Knee Over Knee Twist Stretch

Begin lying on your back, knees bent with one leg crossed over the other and gently pressing in toward the chest. Arms are out to the sides in a T position. Inhale. As you exhale, bring the legs to one side, rotating the hips (1). Keep the legs high into the chest, reaching the top sit bone away from you on a diagonal line from the shoulder. Hold and breathe for 5 to 6 breaths. If the opposite shoulder comes away from the floor, allow it to, and do not force it down. Breathe into the rib cage that is facing the ceiling to stretch the muscles between the ribs, as well as the obliques, outer hip, and low-back muscles. Uncross the legs while you are rotated. Inhaling, bring the top leg back over your chest. Exhaling, bring the other leg back to return to the starting position. Repeat to the other side (2). After you have finished both sides, return to the starting position and roll in small, slow circles on the sacrum a few times in each direction.

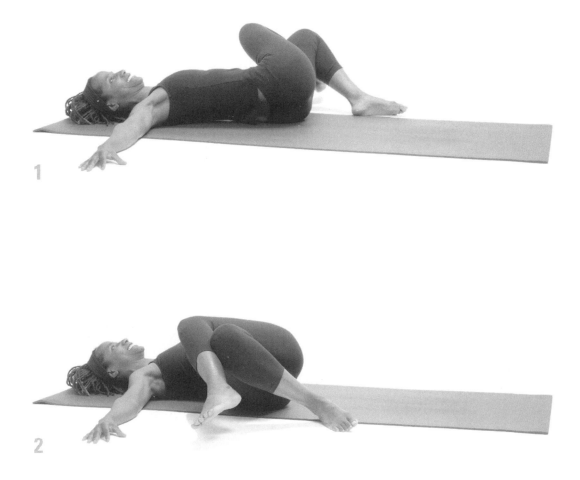

Knee Push-Up

Facing the floor, in a modified plank position, place the arms straight beneath the shoulders perpendicular to the floor. Bend the knees and cross the ankles (1). Form a straight, diagonal line with the head, neck, shoulders, pelvis, and knees. Inhale as you bend the elbows and lower the torso toward the floor (2). As you exhale, straighten the arms and return to the starting position. Distribute your work through the entire body, and be sure the pelvis is in neutral with the head and neck placement in line with the rest of your spine.

Option: Holding this position, breathe in and out for 6 to 8 full breaths.

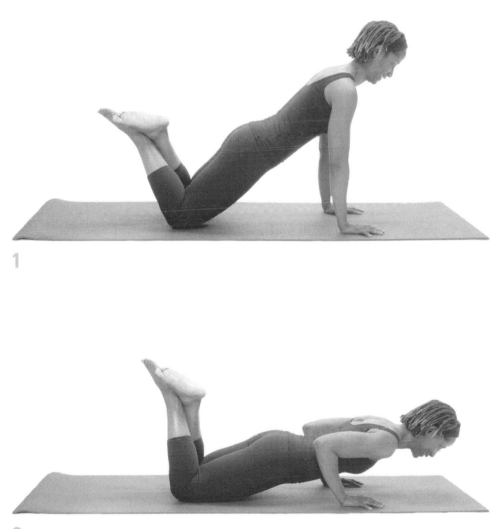

1

2

Leg Circles

Lie on your back with one leg on the floor with the ankle flexed and the other leg reaching to the ceiling, perpendicular to the hip socket, with the foot softly pointed (1). Place the arms in a T position or alongside the torso for a greater challenge. Inhale and exhale one sequence as you anchor the inner unit and pelvis securely in place. As you inhale again, bring the leg in the air slightly across the midline of the torso, keeping the rest of the body stable (2). Exhaling, continue circling the leg down away from you (3), slightly out to the side (4), and back to the starting position. Circle the leg 5 times from the inside and 5 times from the outside. Be sure to keep the pelvis securely anchored in position as the leg rotates in the socket. If the hamstrings are tight, bend the knee of the moving leg. If you feel strain in the lower back, bend the knee of the resting leg and keep the foot flat on the floor.

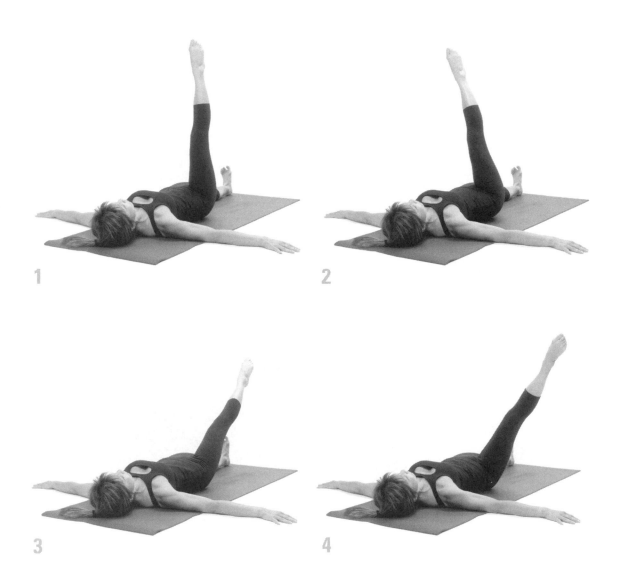

1

2

3

4

Lunge With Hands at Hips

From a kneeling position, bring one foot forward and lunge the torso forward until you feel a stretch in the back leg in the front of the hip joint and top of that thigh. Place the hands at the hips. Keep the back knee down with the top of the foot on the floor. Hold this position to stretch the hip flexors and upper thigh (quadriceps). If the kneecap of the back leg is feeling too much pressure, place a small cushion or towel under it. Hold for 30 to 60 seconds. Keep the pelvis squared with the front edge of the mat and the upper torso in alignment. Repeat to the other side.

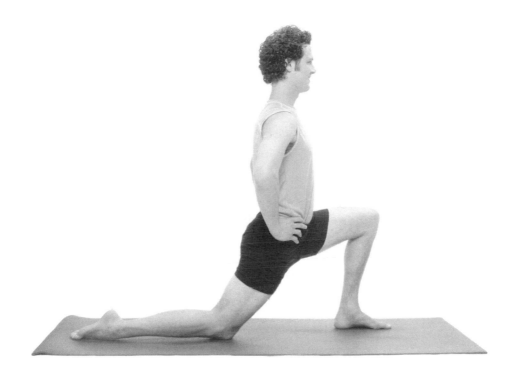

Lunge With Quadriceps Stretch

From a kneeling position, bring one foot forward and lunge the torso forward until you feel a stretch in the back leg at the front of the hip joint and top of that thigh. Place hands at the hips, using the inner thigh muscles of both legs to help keep your balance (1). Be sure to keep your pelvis level with both hip bones square to the front of your mat and avoid rotation.

Reach back with the same arm as the leg behind you and grasp the foot, bending the knee, bringing the foot toward the outer hip and buttock area (2). You may rest the other forearm on your front thigh for support, but do not collapse the body. Bend the back knee only as far as to feel a moderate stretch in the front thigh. Hold for about 60 seconds. Keep the pelvis squared with the front edge of the mat and the upper torso in alignment. Repeat to the other side. If the kneecap of the back leg is feeling too much pressure, a small cushion or towel should be placed underneath it.

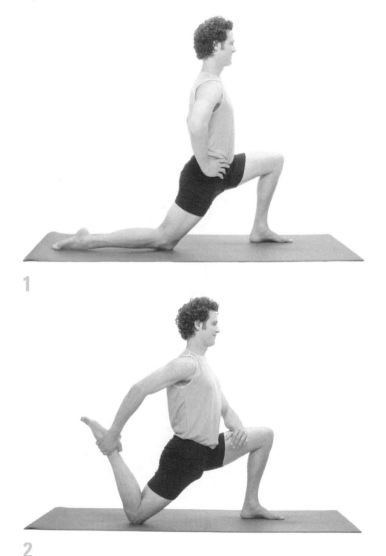

1

2

Neck Pull

Begin lying on your back, with fingers interlaced and placed behind the neck, the outside edge of the pinky finger at the base of the skull (1). Elbows are lifted slightly off of the floor, pointing outward, and legs are straight and pressed together with the ankles flexed. As you inhale, bring the head, neck, and shoulders forward off the floor, keeping the elbows in the same position (2). Avoid pushing the neck or head forward! As you exhale, continue flexing the entire torso forward, articulating through each vertebra of the spine until you cannot curl forward any further (3). Inhaling, bring the torso upright (4). Keep the length through the spine as much as possible. Exhaling, begin to tilt the pelvis back but keep the upper torso lifted (5), and continue to exhale and articulate the spine back to the starting position. Maintain the position of the arms when moving up or down from the floor, and maintain a lengthened sensation throughout the spine even when you are flexing the torso. To decrease difficulty, legs may be slightly apart with ankles flexed or arms may be crossed in front of the chest.

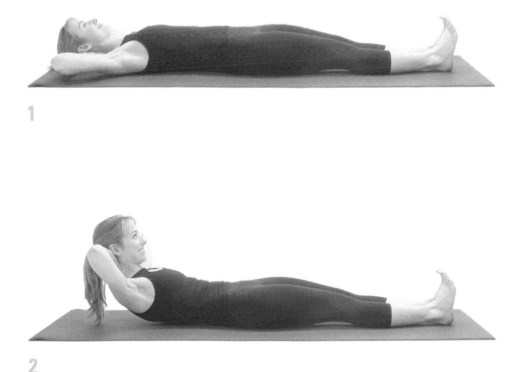

1

2

(continued)

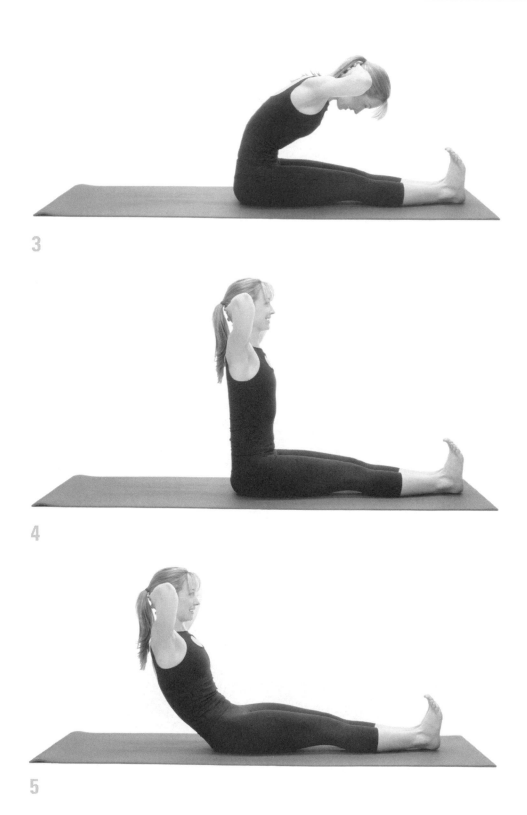

3

4

5

Oblique Rotation

Begin lying on your back, fingers interlaced and placed behind the neck, elbows pointing outward. The right knee is bent toward you, and the left leg is stretched out straight ahead. As you inhale, rotate the torso, bringing the left shoulder toward the right bent knee (1), and exhale as you rotate the right shoulder to the left bent knee (2). As you inhale, again rotate the left shoulder to the right bent knee, and then exhale as you rotate the right shoulder to the left bent knee. Keep the elbows wide so that the rotation is isolated in the trunk and not falsified with simply driving the elbow across the face. Keep the pelvis anchored in neutral.

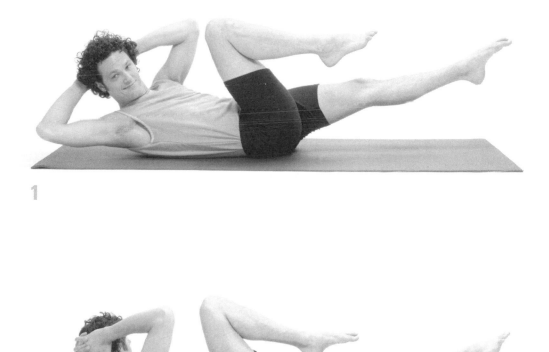

1

2

Open-Leg Rocker

Begin balanced just in back of the tailbone, with the legs straight, shoulder-distance apart, and the hands grasping the top of the ankles (1). Keep arms straight, toes softly pointed, and spine slightly flexed. Inhale. As you exhale, engage the abdominals to roll back to just the upper back (2). Continue exhaling to return to the starting position. It is essential to keep the arms as well as the legs straight throughout the entire movement phase. The spine is slightly flexed to ensure even rolling. Use the abdominals (through the breath) as the impetus for rolling back as well as to brake the upward movement to stop in the starting position. *Never roll onto the neck.*

This exercise is contraindicated for those with preexisting neck problems and those with thoracic osteoporosis.

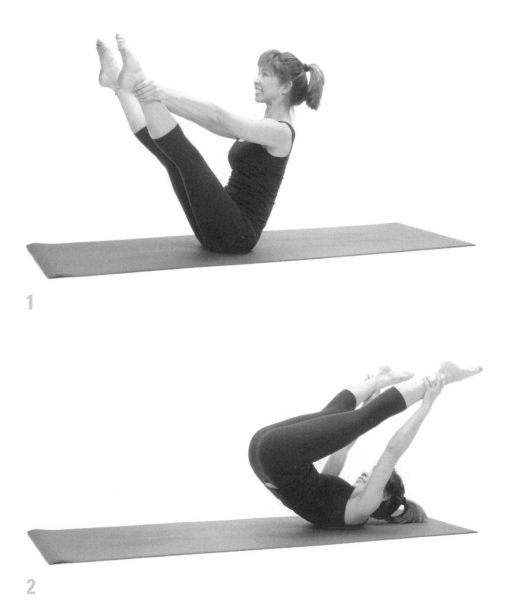

1

2

Pelvic Peel and Hinge

Begin lying on your back with the feet flat on the floor, knees bent, heels in line with the sit bones, and arms next to your trunk with the palms down (1). Place a rolled towel or small ball between the inner thighs. For both variations, use your inner thighs to draw the tailbone away from you when rolling down to feel a tractioning length through the spine. Be sure to coordinate breath with movement.

Peel: Inhale. As you exhale, slowly peel the spine away from the floor starting at the tailbone (2), and articulate through each vertebra until your hips are in a straight, diagonal line with the shoulders and knees (3). Inhale again. As you exhale, begin returning to the starting position from the upper back, articulating through each vertebra using the abdominals. Focus on spinal *articulation* in upward and downward movement.

Hinge: Inhale. As you exhale, bring the pelvis up in one movement and in one piece until it is in a straight diagonal line between the shoulders and knees (3). Inhale again. As you exhale, begin returning to the starting position from the upper back, articulating through each vertebra using the abdominals (4). Focus on pelvic and spinal *stability* in upward movement and spinal *articulation* in downward movement.

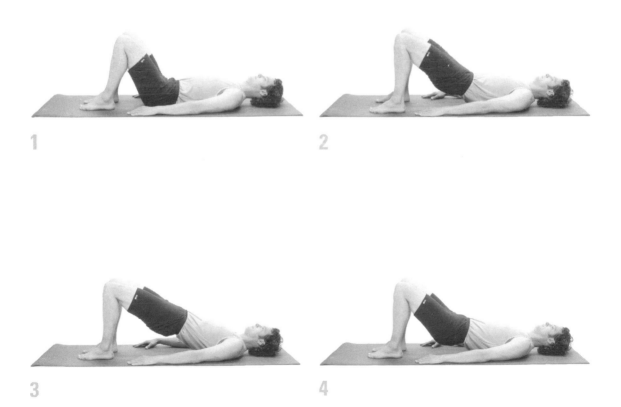

1

2

3

4

Pendulum

Begin lying on your back, legs parallel and pointing toward the ceiling (1). Softly point the toes. Hold the arms out to the sides in a T position or alongside the torso for greater challenge. If the hamstrings are tight, bend the knees. For added support, you can tie a strength band around the legs above the knees. Keep the pelvis neutral. Inhale as the pelvis tips to one side (2). Exhale as you return the pelvis back to center. Repeat to the other side. As in hip rolls, the upper torso should remain stabilized.

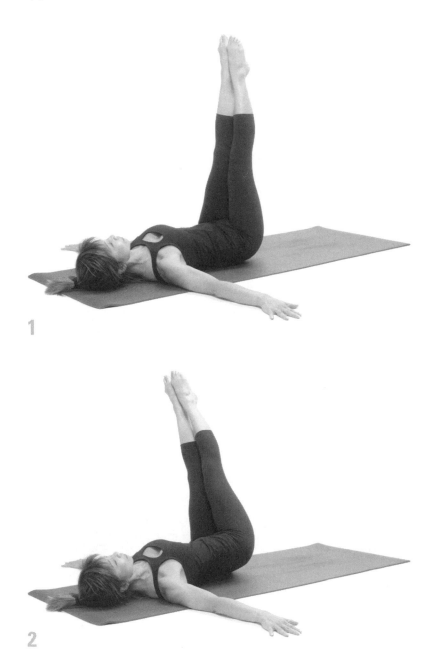

Rolling

Begin balancing just in front of the tailbone with the knees bent into the chest, head down, and arms wrapped around the outside of the shins (1). Feet are not touching the floor. Abdominal connection and shoulder blade stabilization assist you with your balance. Inhale. As you exhale, roll back (2). Exhale more deeply as you roll back up to balance position (double exhalation). Repeat 6 to 8 breaths. Engage the shoulder blades down the back at all times. Be sure you roll only onto the upper back, never onto your neck. It is important to feel the use of the abdominals as the impetus for rolling back, as well as to brake the upward movement to stop in the starting position. Maintain the ball shape throughout the rolling phase.

This exercise is contraindicated for those participants with thoracic osteoporosis or pre-existing neck issues.

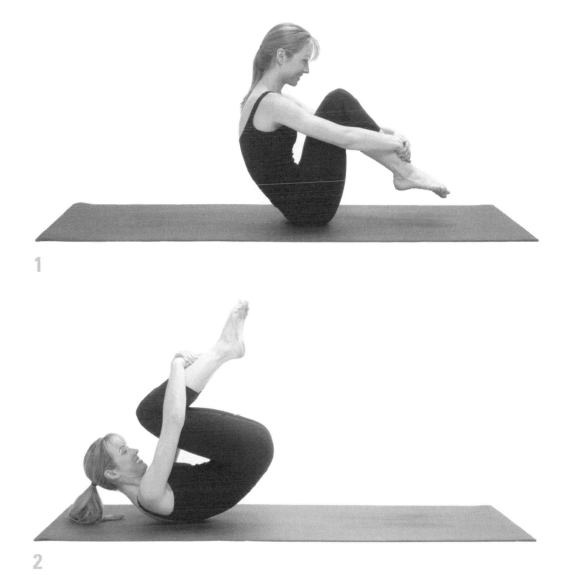

1

2

Rollover

Begin lying on your back with your arms at your sides, palms down, and legs together and reaching to the ceiling with the feet softly pointed (1). If the hamstrings are tight, you may slightly bend the knees. Inhale. As you exhale, begin rolling the pelvis back using the abdominals as you curl the spine (tail end) toward you. Your legs will begin to reach toward your head into a modified plow position (2). Inhale as you open the legs shoulder-distance apart and flex the ankles (3). As you exhale, begin articulating the spine sequentially one vertebra at a time back toward the floor with control keeping the legs apart (4). Return to the starting position. Inhale as you bring the legs together using the inner thighs, and point the feet. Exhale, and repeat the movements. Repeat 5 times, then repeat 5 more times initiating the rollover with the legs apart. Be sure to "ride the wave of the breath" so that all movements are smooth and controlled. If the hamstrings are tight, be sure to bend the knees.

This exercise is contraindicated for those individuals with thoracic osteoporosis and preexisting neck problems.

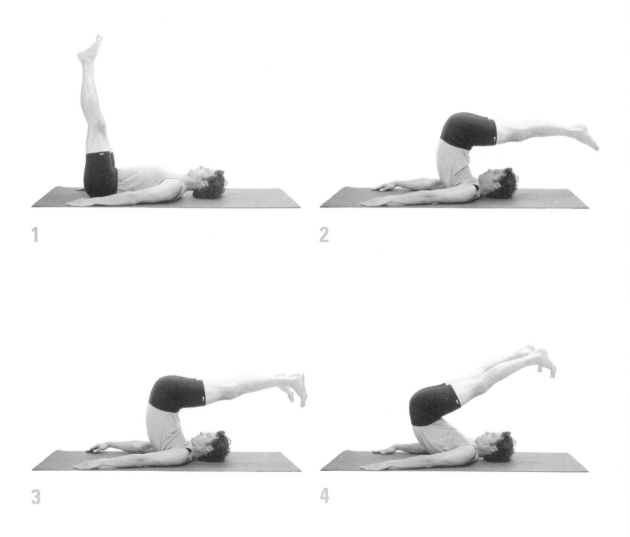

1

2

3

4

Begin lying on your back with the legs together, parallel, and the ankles flexed (1). Arms are reaching overhead alongside the ears with the palms toward one another. Inhaling, bring the arms up perpendicular to the floor and curl the upper torso forward, bringing the head in between the frame formed by the arms. Exhaling, lower the arms over the legs, and engage the abdominals to smoothly articulate the spine upward (2) until you are reaching the arms long over the legs parallel to the floor (3). Inhale in this position, and exhale as you articulate the spine one vertebra at a time back down to the starting position. Be sure to keep the shoulder blades anchored on the back and avoid hunching the shoulders. Work as smoothly as possible, using the breath to assist in controlling the movements.

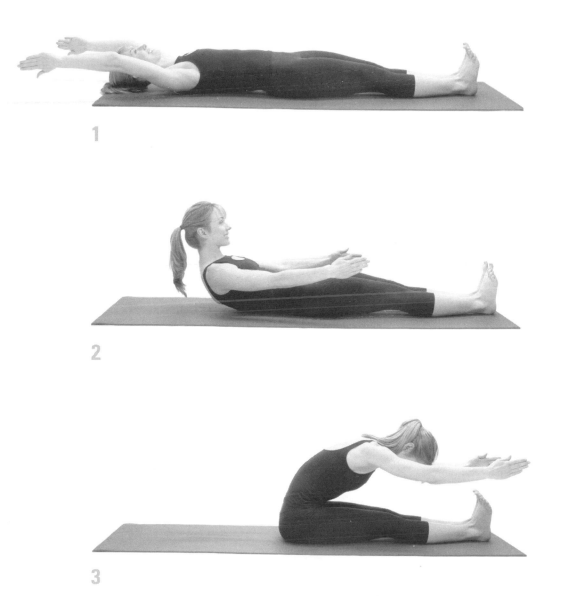

1

2

3

Roll-Up With Strength Band and Shoulder Rotation

Begin lying on your back, legs apart and the ankles flexed (1). Arms are reaching overhead alongside the ears and holding the strength band with light tension between the hands. Inhaling, bring arms upward, perpendicular to the floor, keeping the band taut (2), and curl the upper torso forward while bringing the head in between the frame formed by the arms. Exhaling, lower arms over legs and engage the abdominals to smoothly articulate the spine upward until arms are parallel to the floor (3). Inhaling, sit upright and rotate the arms up (4) and then behind you, stretching open the chest and shoulders, stretching the band if needed (5). Exhale as the arms continue down behind you. Inhaling, bring the arms back up and around to the front and flex the spine forward, arms again parallel to the floor (3). Exhaling, articulate the spine one vertebra at a time back down to the starting position. Keep the shoulder blades anchored on the back as you go through the arm movement and chest stretch. Perform this exercise with the legs together for a greater challenge.

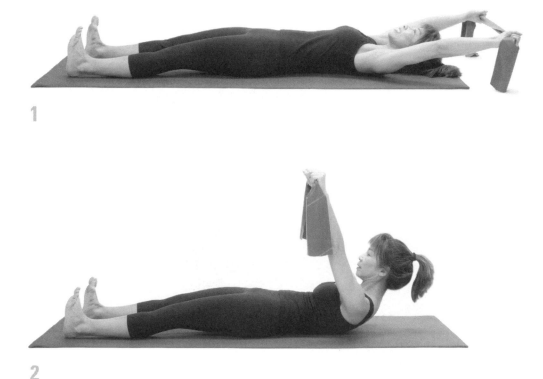

1

2

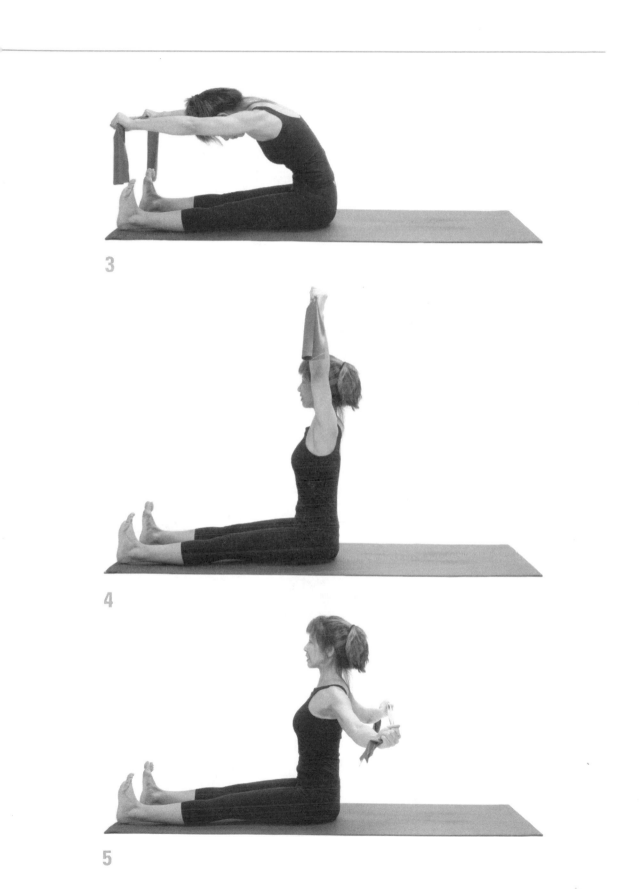

3

4

5

Saw

Begin seated upright with your pelvis in the neutral position, legs apart slightly wider than shoulder distance, and ankles flexed (1). Leg muscles are fully engaged at all times. Arms are out to the sides, at shoulder height. Engage the inner unit. Inhaling, rotate the torso to the left (2). Keep the pelvis stable. Exhaling, flex the torso forward, reaching the right hand toward the left foot (3). Look toward the back arm if possible; if the neck feels strained, look toward the front hand. Inhale, bringing the torso back up still rotated to the left (2). Exhale as you return the torso back to the starting position. As an added option, you may add a double pulse when the hand is reaching toward the foot. Repeat to the other side.

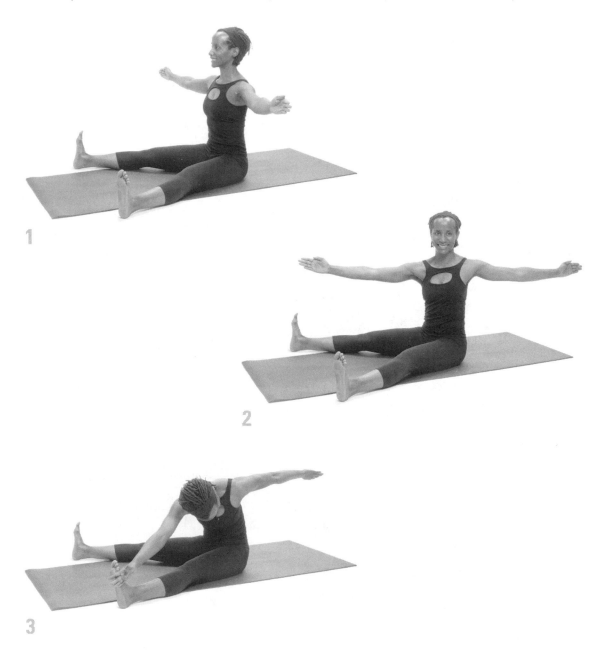

Saw With Back Extension

Begin seated upright with your pelvis in the neutral position, legs apart slightly wider than shoulder distance, and ankles flexed (1). Leg muscles are fully engaged at all times. Arms are out to the sides, at shoulder height. Engage the inner unit. Inhaling, rotate the torso to the left (2). Keep the pelvis stable. Exhaling, flex the torso forward, reaching the right hand toward the left foot (3). Look toward the back arm if possible; if the neck feels strained, look toward the front hand. Inhale as you bring the torso back up, still rotated to the left and arch back, lifting the chest (spine extension), leaning slightly back on the left hand (4). Feel a tension connection from the lower ribs to the sacral base to support the lumbar spine. As you exhale, return the torso back upright and to the starting position. Repeat to the other side.

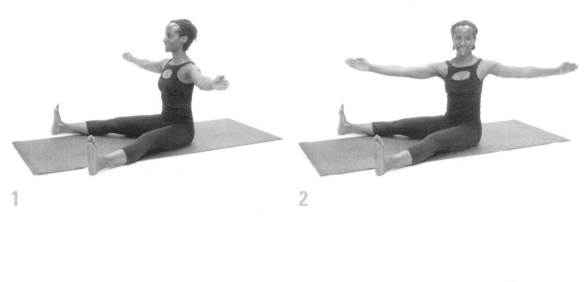

1

2

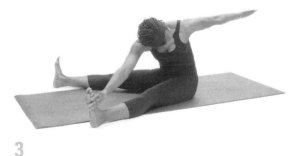

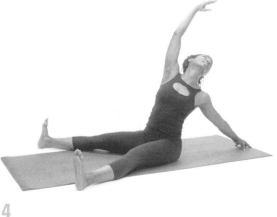

3

4

Scissors

Begin lying on your back, pelvis neutral. Bring one leg toward the torso with the hands grasping the back of the leg (1). Keep the leg straight! Reach the other leg long and away, bringing it to about a 45-degree angle or lower if you have no back strain. Fully engage muscles of both legs. As you inhale, perform a scissor action with the legs, switching their position as well as hand hold (2). As you exhale, scissor the legs while you switch again. Pelvis must remain in neutral position! When switching legs, keep them fairly close together. You can further challenge respiratory strength by inhaling for two changes and exhaling for two changes.

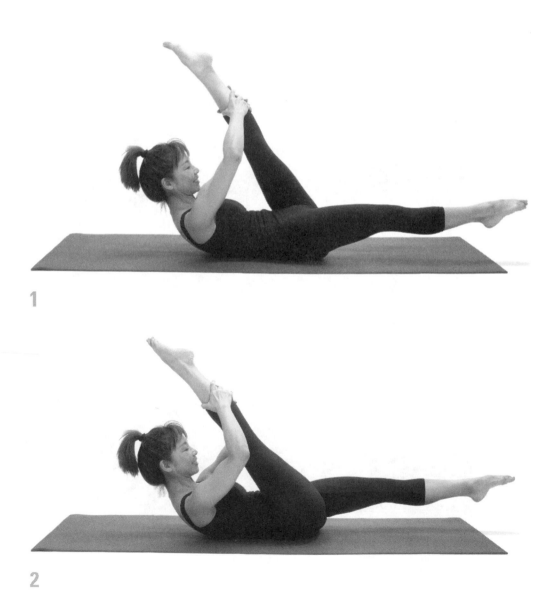

1

2

Seal

Seated upright, bend knees, and fold the legs toward the torso with the knees opened to the sides. Reach both arms to the inside of the legs and grasp the outside of each ankle with the same-side hand (1). Bring the feet up so that they are approximately in front of the navel. Slightly flex the spine using the abdominals without collapsing the chest so that you can balance just behind the tailbone and in front of the sit bones. Inhaling clap the feet together twice. Exhaling, roll back (2), and continue to exhale as you roll back up to the starting position. Roll from the tailbone to the top of the upper back only, never onto the neck. Keep the spine curved at all times, and use the abdominals to create the movement back as well as to brake the movement when returning upright. You must engage the pelvic floor at all times.

This exercise is contraindicated for those participants with thoracic osteoporosis or pre-existing neck issues.

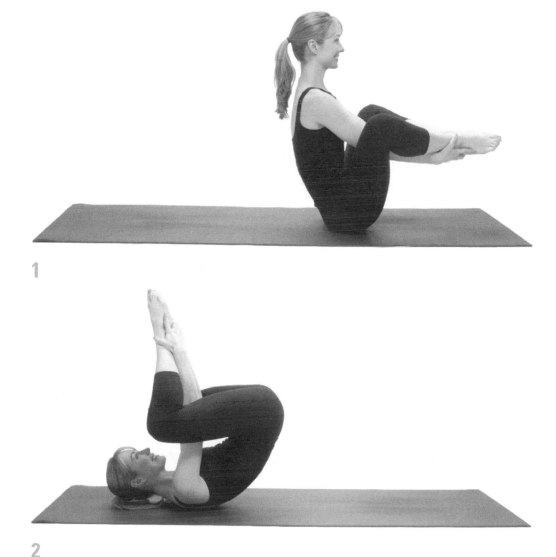

1

2

Seated Hip Stretch

Seated upright, cross one leg over the other in a figure 4 position. Top leg is bent at the knee, with the outside ankle bone just above the opposite knee and outside the thigh. The top leg's knee will be to the outside of torso. Ankle is flexed. Place your hands slightly behind the torso and lean back with a neutral spine and pelvis. Chest stays lifted. Draw the bottom leg up toward you, keeping the top leg placed so that the knee is kept to the outside. You will begin to feel a stretch in the outside hip area of the top leg. Bring the leg in as close as possible while maintaining a neutral pelvis. Avoid allowing the spine to collapse back. If you have low-back problems, you may recline and opt for the figure 4 stretch in chapter 4, page 63.

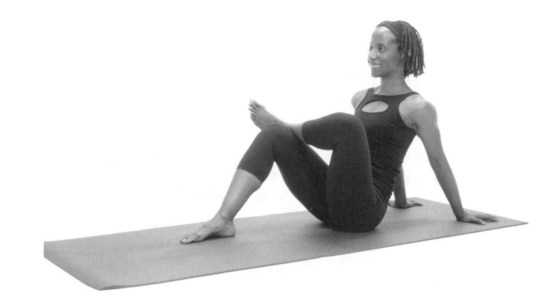

Seated Shoulder Stretch

Seated upright, grasp a strength band slightly wider than shoulder-width apart with the arms lowered in front of the torso (1). Maintain some tension between the hands, but do not pull. Arms are straight but not locked. Legs are in any position that is comfortable (usually I bend them to cross-legged position) as long as the pelvis stays neutral. Inhaling, bring the arms up in front of you and keep them straight (2). Exhaling, continue to rotate the arms (shoulders) all the way around behind you, feeling a strong stretch in the front of the chest near the shoulders (3). Keep the shoulder blades down! Inhale as you bring the arms up from behind you to above the head again (2). Exhale as you bring the arms back down the front of the torso to the starting position (1). Head and neck should not have to shift for the arms to complete the circle. If you experience strain in the shoulders or neck area, widen the grip between the hands.

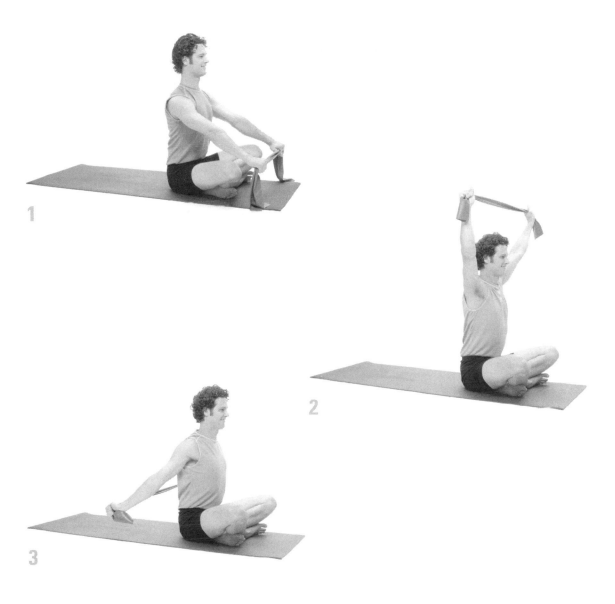

1

2

3

Shoulder Bridge With Leg Pulse

Begin lying on your back, knees bent at 90 degrees. Shins are perpendicular to the floor, heels positioned directly below the knees and in the line with the sit bones (1). Arms are bent at the elbow and the hands are supporting the lower back. Position the elbows directly below the wrists. (If wrist position is uncomfortable, lace fingers and keep arms on the floor under your hips or simply rest the arms flat on the floor.) Roll the front of the chest open at the shoulders as much as possible. Inhaling, bring your right leg up toward the ceiling and gently double-pulse it toward your torso with the ankle flexed (2). Exhaling, bring the leg toward the floor with control using the hamstrings and glutes, pointing the foot (3). Repeat with the same leg 3 times, and then change sides. Be sure that the pelvis stays steady at all times. Engage the inner thighs to avoid letting the legs stray open to the side.

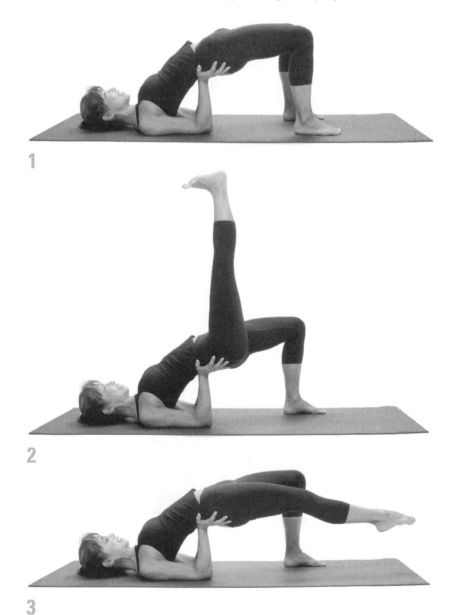

1

2

3

Side Bend

Begin seated sideways, the top leg bent at the knee and the sole of that foot flat on the floor (1). Bottom leg is also bent at the knee with the side of the leg resting on the floor. Hand of the bottom arm is placed flat on the floor just slightly wider than the shoulder, fingers pointing away from the torso. Top arm is resting on the top knee with the palm up. Inhaling, straighten the legs and lift the hips up in the air (2). Legs press together with the inner thigh muscles. Top arm sweeps in a large arc over the head. The shoulder of the weight-bearing arm must be strongly stabilized using the scapular stabilizers. Reach the hips upward so that the torso, legs, and arm assume the shape of a large crescent. Use the muscles in the hip on the side that is toward the floor to assist in elevating the height of the hips, and engage the leg muscles. Exhaling, return the legs, arm, and torso back to the starting position with control.

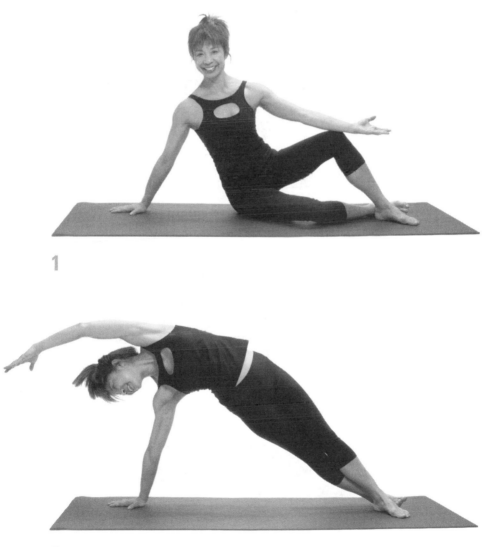

1

2

Side Kick, Propped on Elbow

Begin lying on your side with both legs straight and angled at the hip about 20 degrees in front of you. Both ankles are flexed. The bottom arm is bent at the elbow with the hand placed alongside the head, and the lower triceps area just above the elbow is anchored to the floor. The top hand is placed on the floor in front of the chest to assist in balance. The entire underside of the torso is off the floor and forms one straight line from head to pelvis. Strongly engage the T point (located straight back to the spine from the lowest point of your breastbone) to avoid flaring the rib cage. Inhaling, bring the top leg parallel to the floor, reaching long out of the hip with the foot pointed (1). Exhaling, maintain this position with the deep abdominals and back muscles. Inhaling, bring the top leg forward, flexing at the hip, and pulse the leg twice (2). Exhaling, point the foot and carry the leg back behind the hips, only as far as possible while still maintaining the stability of the torso and pelvis (3). Be sure to keep the top leg parallel with the floor at all times, and avoid letting it drift up and down in height.

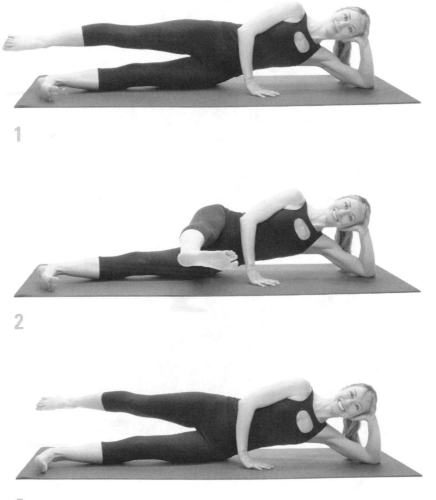

1

2

3

Single-Leg Stretch

Begin lying on your back with the pelvis in neutral and the upper torso flexed forward. Bring one knee toward the chest with the outside hand placed at the ankle and the inside hand placed at the same knee (1). Reach the other leg long into the distance, bringing it to about a 45-degree angle or lower if you have no back strain. Inhale as you switch legs, changing hand position as well (2). Exhale as you switch leg and hand position again. Be sure to keep the elbows wide with the shoulders down. It is hand over hand to change hand position with the leg switch. Repeat, maintaining your neutral pelvis. You can further challenge respiratory strength by inhaling for two changes and exhaling for two changes.

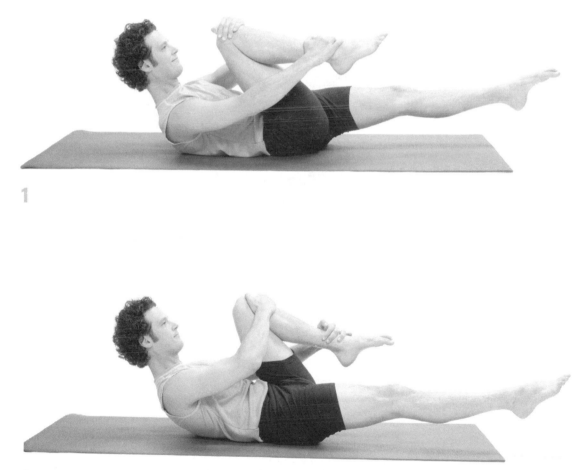

1

2

Spine Spiral With Double Pulse

Begin seated upright, legs crossed (1). Arms are in front of the chest at shoulder height with the elbows bent and fingertips touching. Torso is in upright neutral position. Inhaling, rotate the upper torso to the right and straighten the right elbow (2). Begin your rotation from the lower ribs. As you rotate the torso, imagine you are spiraling upward. Gently pulse to the right twice using the obliques. Use the leverage of the pulsing arm to assist in deepening the spiral. Be aware to avoid jerking the arm when straightening the elbow. As you exhale, rotate the torso back to starting position, returning the arm back to the starting position while keeping the spine uplifted. Repeat to the other side.

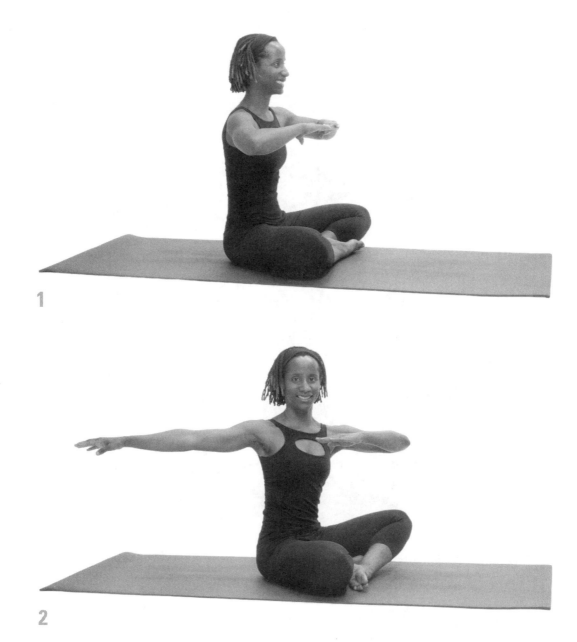

1

2

Spine Stretch With Extension

Begin sitting upright with the legs stretched in front of you straight and opened to approximately 90 degrees with the ankles flexed (1). Bend the knees if hamstring shortness prevents an upright, neutral pelvis. Stretch the arms in front of you, parallel to the floor, at shoulder height with the palms down. Inhale to prepare and lengthen the spine. As you exhale, flex the spine forward until the fingertips touch the floor (2). Inhale in this position. Exhaling, slide the fingers forward, increasing the flexion of the spine. Avoid collapsing in the chest and shoulders. Inhale in the flexed spine position. As you exhale, return the spine, vertebra by vertebra, to the starting position (1). Inhale as you place the hands on the floor behind the hips (3) and arch the upper torso slightly back (spinal extension). Exhale as you return to the starting position.

1

2

3

Spine Twist With Arms Moving Upward

Begin seated upright with legs stretched straight in front of you, parallel and together, and ankles flexed (1). Arms are out to the sides, palms facing forward. Inhaling, rotate the upper torso to the left, reaching both arms upward alongside the ears with the palms facing toward the head (2). Imagine you are spiraling upward as you rotate the torso. Scapulae should be stabilized on the back so that the upper shoulder and neck area does not elevate or tense when moving the arms. Exhaling, begin to rotate the torso back to the starting position, returning the arms back to the starting position. Maintain the uplifted spine when rotating back to the front. Repeat to the other side.

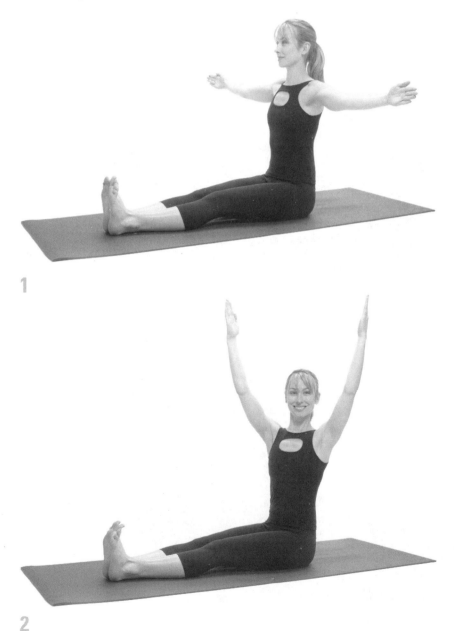

1

2

Spine Twist With Lat Pull

Begin seated upright with legs stretched straight in front of you, parallel and pressed together, and ankles flexed (1). Arms are grasping a strength band with hands slightly wider than shoulders and held overhead. Inhaling, rotate the upper torso to the left, pulling the strength band down to the upper chest using the lats (2). Begin your rotation from the lower ribs. Imagine you are spiraling upward as you rotate the torso, and feel the rotation of the upper arm bones in the shoulder sockets. Don't lose your T point (located straight back to the spine from the lowest point of the breastbone) when pulling the band downward toward the chest. Exhaling, rotate the torso back to center, returning the arms up to the overhead position. Maintain the uplifted sensation in the spine. Repeat to the other side.

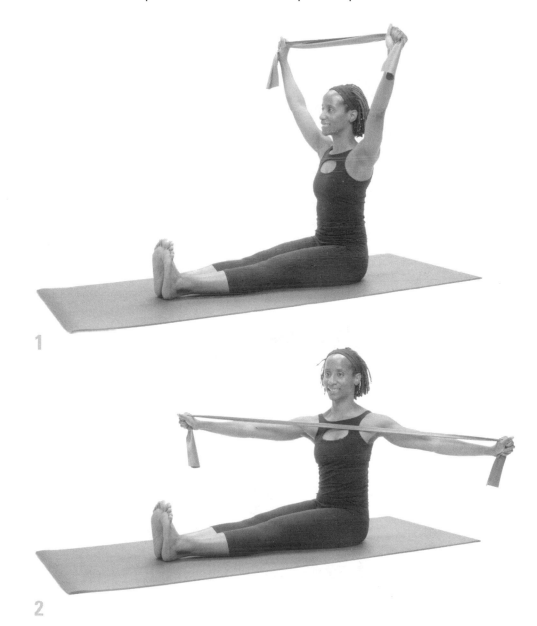

1

2

Swan (Modified Rocking)

Begin lying on your front, elbows bent, hands placed flat near the shoulders, elbows pointing toward the legs (1). Legs reach behind you, straight, slightly turned out, approximately 6 to 8 inches (15 to 20 centimeters) apart. Inhale and bring the upper trunk into extension via the back muscles with some assistance from the arms (2). Be sure that the legs are engaged and reaching long out of the hips. Exhaling, "dive" the torso toward the floor (3) as the arms immediately reach to the side (less shoulder flexibility) or forward (more shoulder flexibility). Use the momentum to assist the diving movement as well as the strength of the legs reaching out and upward into extension ("lift your tail feathers"). Inhaling, immediately fold the arms so that the palms are again in the starting position to assist in the upper trunk extension, and repeat movements. The energy and distribution of work should reach through the entire body at all times. Timing and coordination of the arms returning under the shoulders is crucial for execution.

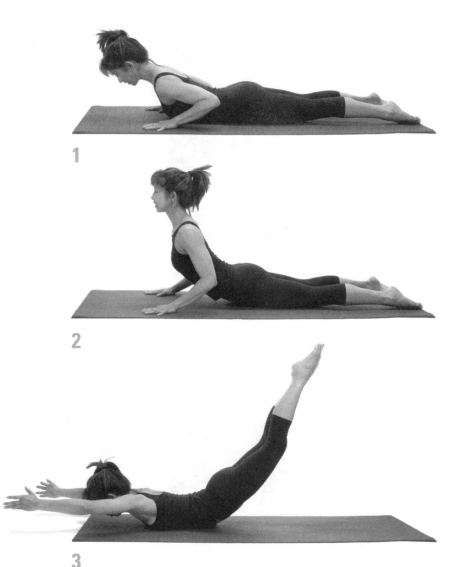

1

2

3

Swimming

Begin lying on your front with the arms and legs reaching in opposite directions. Keep the legs parallel, heels in line with the sitting bones. The face and chest are hovering off the floor, and the head and neck are aligned with the rest of the spine. Inhaling, move the opposing arm and leg slightly higher away from the floor in a swimming motion for four movements (1). Exhaling, repeat again, moving the opposing arm and leg for four movements (2). Be sure to reach the arm and leg off the floor only as far as you can without disturbing the stability of your pelvis and shoulder girdle.

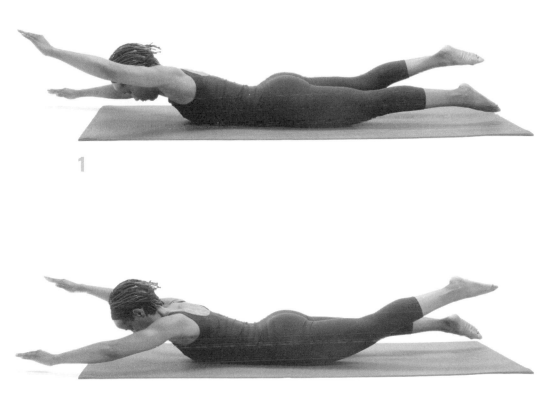

1

2

Twist

Begin seated sideways with the top leg bent at the knee and the sole of that foot flat on the floor (1). The bottom leg is also bent at the knee with the side of the leg resting on the floor. Feet are placed near one another. The hand of the bottom arm is placed flat on the floor slightly wider than the shoulder, and fingers are pointing away from the torso. The top arm is resting on the top knee with the palm facing up. Inhaling, straighten the legs while pressing them together as you lift the hips up and bring the top arm up to a letter T position (2). Exhaling, rotate the torso toward the floor, hinge the weight of the torso onto the legs, and reach the top arms around the torso underneath the supporting arm (3). The legs should be strong and engaged as much as possible. Move the head to look toward the reaching hand. You must engage the shoulder girdle stabilizers, especially on the weight-bearing arm. Inhaling, return the arm and torso to the diagonally neutral position with the top arm again in the T position (2). Exhaling, return back down to the floor.

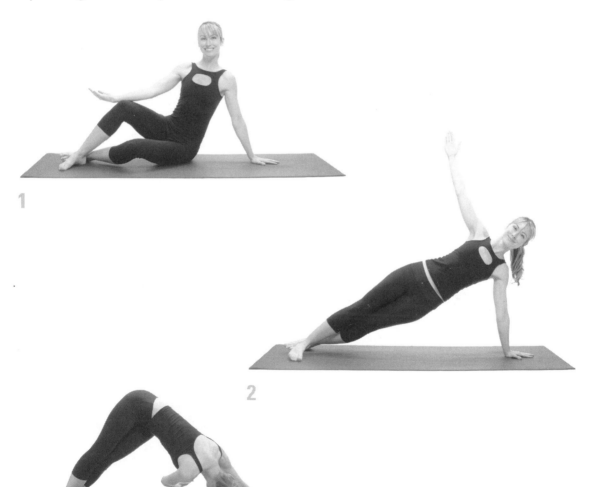

1

2

3

6

Intense Workouts

20-Minute Intense Workout

The 20-minute intense routine will definitely give you the shorter but challenging all-around quickie you are looking for. Included are balance and timing challenges such as the boomerang and an advanced side kick variation. This routine is shorter in time, but it gives you a charge that lasts the whole day. Try focusing on breath control to intenify the experience.

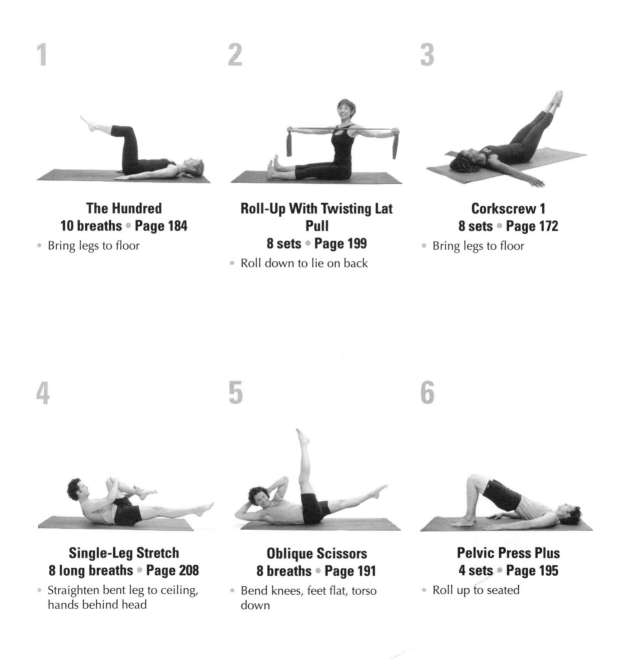

1

The Hundred
10 breaths • Page 184

* Bring legs to floor

2

Roll-Up With Twisting Lat Pull
8 sets • Page 199

* Roll down to lie on back

3

Corkscrew 1
8 sets • Page 172

* Bring legs to floor

4

Single-Leg Stretch
8 long breaths • Page 208

* Straighten bent leg to ceiling, hands behind head

5

Oblique Scissors
8 breaths • Page 191

* Bend knees, feet flat, torso down

6

Pelvic Press Plus
4 sets • Page 195

* Roll up to seated

7

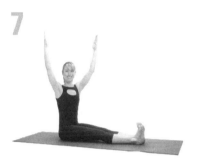

Spine Spiral With Arms Up
6 sets • Page 209

- Open legs to V position

8

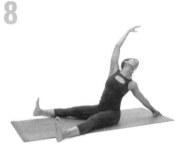

Saw With Back Extension
5 sets • Page 200

- Bring legs up to open V position, grasp ankles

9

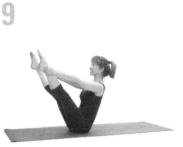

Open-Leg Rocker
6 sets • Page 192

- Bring legs to floor, sit upright

10

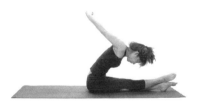

Boomerang
6 sets • Page 166

- Bend knees, cross ankles, move to plank

11

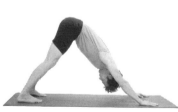

Downward Dog
3 breaths • Page 177

- Step one leg forward

12

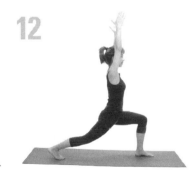

Lunge (Standing)
30 to 60 seconds on each leg
Page 186

- Step into plank, lower torso to floor

(continued)

13

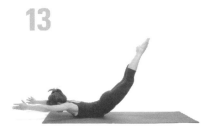

Swan (Rocking)
8 breaths • Page 211

- Sweep arms to behind back, turn head

14

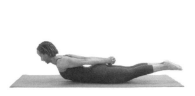

Double-Leg Kick
8 sets • Page 175

- Turn to lie on one side

15

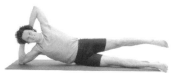

Side Kick With Bent Elbows
8 sets each side • Page 206

- Sit up sideways

16

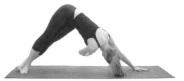

Twist
6 sets • Page 214

- Rotate to plank and lower torso to floor

17

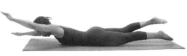

Swimming
8 breaths • Page 212

- Roll over onto your back and sit up

18

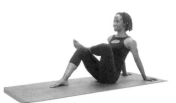

Seated Hip Stretch
30 to 60 seconds per side
Page 203

- Stretch arms and legs out and lie on back

19

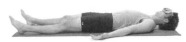

Corpse
Relax 1 minute • Page 174

40-Minute Intense Workout

The 40-minute intense workout will definitely challenge you in the morning. Included are the classic versions of hip circles, side kick (kneeling), and rocking bow. There are also upper-body challenges with mermaid and back support. Exercises that involve flexibility and strength, as well as coordination, timing, and balance give this jam packed routine a punch that is sure to leave you energized and raring to go!

1

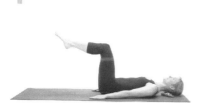

The Hundred
10 breaths • Page 184

- Bend knees, place feet on floor

2

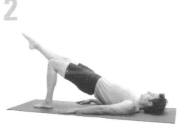

Pelvic Peel With Leg Abduction and Adduction
4 to 6 sets • Page 194

- Straighten legs, bring arms overhead by ears

3

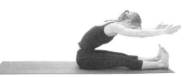

Roll-Up (Advanced)
8 sets • Page 198

- Bring legs to reach up to ceiling

4

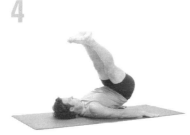

Corkscrew 2
5 sets • Page 173

- Roll up to seated and open legs

5

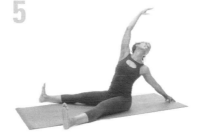

Saw With Back Extension
6 sets • Page 200

- Bring legs up in air, grasp ankles

6

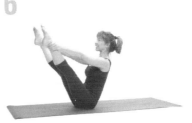

Open-Leg Rocker
8 sets • Page 192

- Close legs, arms reach to feet

7

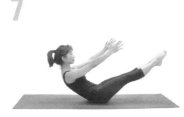

Teaser
8 sets • Page 213

- Lower legs, cross at ankles

8

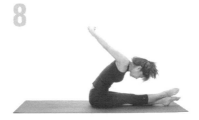

Boomerang
8 sets • Page 166

- Bring legs up in parallel to 45 degrees

9

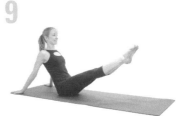

Hip Circles
6 sets • Page 183

- Lower legs to floor

(continued)

10

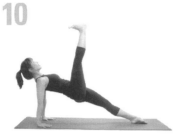

Back Support
6 sets • Page 164
- Tuck legs in a side sitting position

11

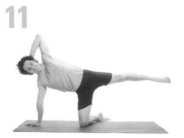

Side Kick (Kneeling)
8 sets per side • Page 205
- Bring hips down to a side sitting position

12

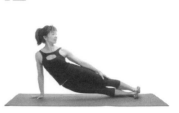

Mermaid
5 sets per side • Page 187
- Turn toward floor into a plank position

13

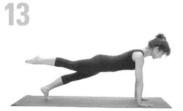

Front Support With Push-Ups
8 sets • Page 181
- Lower torso to floor

14

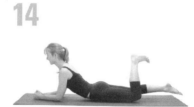

Single-Leg Kick (Advanced)
8 sets • Page 207
- Lower upper torso, turn head, hands behind back

15

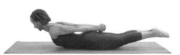

Double-Leg Kick
8 sets • Page 175
- Place hands at shoulders, press hips up and back

16

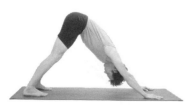

Downward Dog
1 to 2 breaths • Page 177
- Move torso forward to plank, turn to side sitting

17

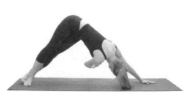

Twist
6 sets • Page 214
- Turn onto back, bend knees, feet flat

18

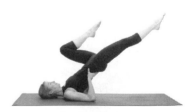

Bicycle
5 sets each direction
Page 165
- Same position

19

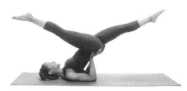

Bridging Scissors
8 sets • Page 169

- Lower hips, roll up to seated position

20

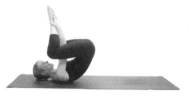

Seal (Advanced)
6 sets • Page 202

- Turn to side sitting position

21

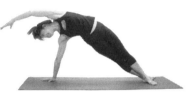

Side Bend
6 sets per side • Page 204

- Turn to floor and lie down

22

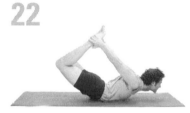

Bow (Rocking)
6 to 8 sets • Page 168

- Come to hands and knees

23

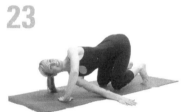

Cat Twist
4 sets • Page 170

- Turn to lie on back

24

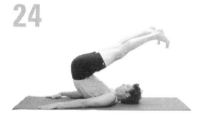

Rollover
4 sets each direction
Page 197

- Same position

25

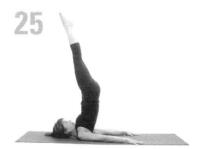

Jackknife
5 sets • Page 185

- Bend knees to chest and roll over to front

26

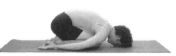

Child's Pose
30 to 60 seconds • Page 171

- Bring body upright to seated

27

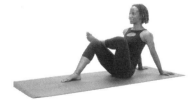

Seated Hip Stretch
30 to 60 seconds per side
Page 203

60-Minute Intense Workout

Go for the gold! This is the most challenging workout routine offered in this series. Since you have chosen this level of intensity and duration, you will attain even more from your effort if you can move from exercise to exercise smoothly with the transitions described. Not only will you gain coordination benefits, but your mental acuity will be honed to an even more refined level. Congratulations on making this your morning routine of choice. Remember to engage your inner unit as you move from exercise to exercise. *Breathe so that you can concentrate on your center to control the precise flowing movements!*

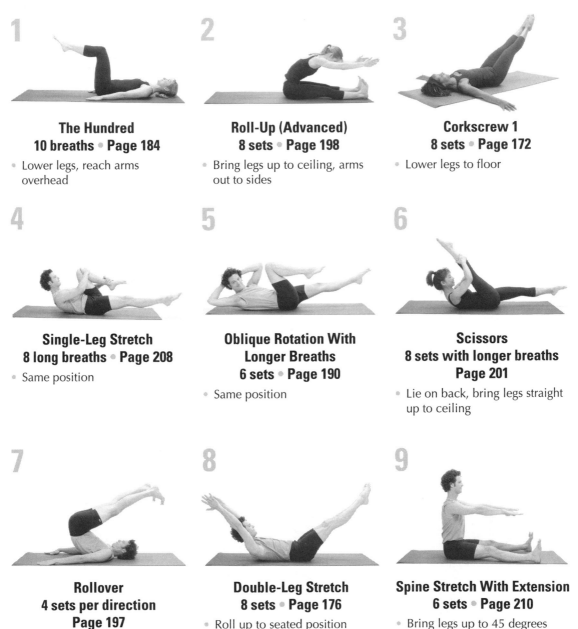

1

The Hundred
10 breaths • Page 184

• Lower legs, reach arms overhead

2

Roll-Up (Advanced)
8 sets • Page 198

• Bring legs up to ceiling, arms out to sides

3

Corkscrew 1
8 sets • Page 172

• Lower legs to floor

4

Single-Leg Stretch
8 long breaths • Page 208

• Same position

5

Oblique Rotation With Longer Breaths
6 sets • Page 190

• Same position

6

Scissors
8 sets with longer breaths
Page 201

• Lie on back, bring legs straight up to ceiling

7

Rollover
4 sets per direction
Page 197

• Bring legs to floor

8

Double-Leg Stretch
8 sets • Page 176

• Roll up to seated position

9

Spine Stretch With Extension
6 sets • Page 210

• Bring legs up to 45 degrees

10

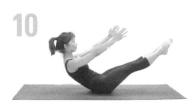

Teaser
8 sets • Page 213

• Lower legs to floor and open

11

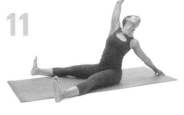

Saw With Back Extension
6 sets • Page 200

• Bring legs up, open, and grasp ankles

12

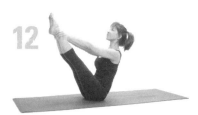

Open and Close Leg Rocker
5 sets • Page 193

• Close legs, place hands behind hips

13

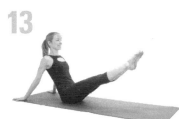

Hip Circles
8 sets • Page 183

• Roll down, bring legs over to plow position

14

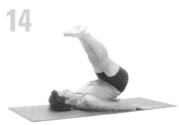

Corkscrew 2
6 sets • Page 173

• Lower legs, roll up to seated position

15

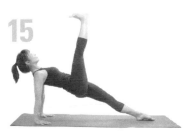

Back Support
6 sets • Page 164

• Bend knees, cross ankles, step back to plank

16

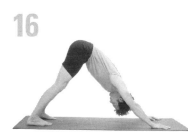

Downward Dog
1 to 2 breaths • Page 177

• Step one foot forward

17

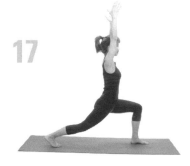

Lunge (Standing)
30 to 60 seconds per leg
Page 186

• Step to plank, lower torso

18

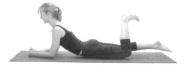

Single-Leg Kick (Advanced)
8 sets • Page 207

• Press up to plank

(continued)

19

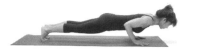

Front Support With Downward Dog and Push-Up
8 cycles each exercise
Page 179

- Lower torso to floor

20

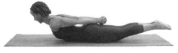

Double-Leg Kick
8 sets • Page 175

- Hold final extension, sweep arms around to head

21

Swimming
8 breaths • Page 212

- Press to child's pose, turn to side sitting

22

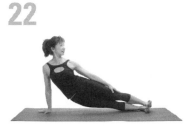

Mermaid
6 sets to one side • Page 187

- Turn to rest on front on the floor

23

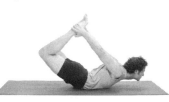

Bow (Rocking)
6 to 8 sets • Page 168

- Child's pose into side sitting

24

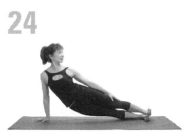

Mermaid
6 sets to other side
Page 187

- Turn to rest on front on the floor

25

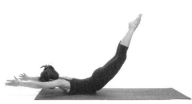

Swan (Rocking)
8 breaths • Page 211

- Turn to side sitting position

26

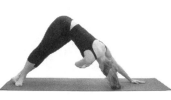

Twist
6 sets • Page 214

- Roll onto back with legs to ceiling

27

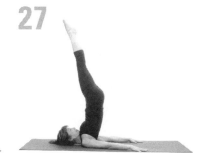

Jackknife
5 sets • Page 185

- Bend knees, place feet flat on floor

28

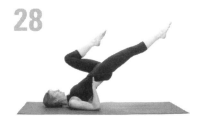

**Bicycle
5 sets each direction
Page 165**

• Same position

29

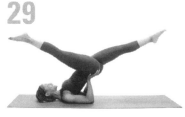

**Bridging Scissors
8 sets • Page 169**

• Lower legs and hips to floor

30

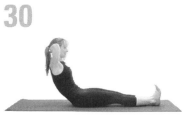

**Neck Pull
5 sets • Page 188**

• Last rep, remain seated upright

31

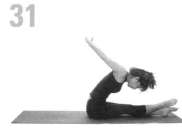

**Boomerang
8 sets • Page 166**

• Roll back to lying on floor

32

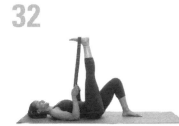

**Hamstring and Inner Thigh
Stretch With Band
30 to 60 seconds per stretch
per leg • Page 182**

• Same position

33

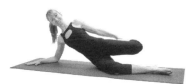

**Figure 4 Stretch
30 to 60 seconds per side
Page 178**

• Roll to side

34

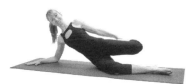

**Quad Release
30 to 60 seconds per leg
Page 196**

Back Support

From a seated position with the legs together and the hands placed behind the hips, lift your pelvis until it is in one straight line between the shoulders and feet (1). Keep the head and neck in line with the rest of the spine. Inhaling, bring the right leg straight up with a flexed ankle and pulse gently twice (2). Distribute the workload throughout the entire body so that you don't overly fatigue the arms and shoulders. Press the soles of the feet into the floor as much as possible. If the calves cramp from lack of ankle flexibility, keep the heels in strong contact with the floor to engage the entire back of the legs. Press the inner thighs firmly together as well. Exhaling, return the right leg back to the starting position. Inhaling, bring the left leg up with the ankle flexed and pulse gently twice. Exhaling, return the left leg back to the starting position. Maintain height and stability of the pelvis at all times.

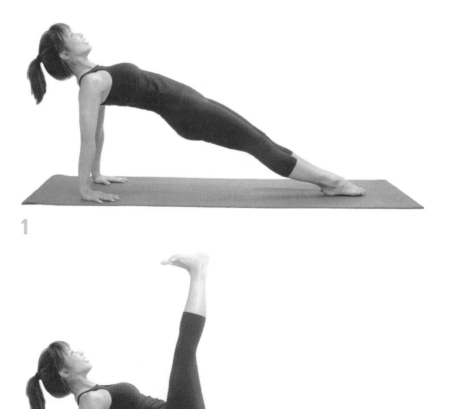

1

2

Bicycle

Begin lying on your back with both hands under the lower back. Forearms are perpendicular to the floor and shoulders are rolled underneath you (1). One leg is bent at the knee toward the chest and the other leg is extended away from the torso (legs look as though they are lunging). Feet are pointed. Inhaling, extend the bent knee toward the ceiling (2) and bring the leg down away from you while simultaneously bending the other knee and bringing it in toward the torso (bicycling legs). Exhaling, repeat the movement. Keep the movement smooth while engaging the deep abdominals to support the spine and maintain torso stability. Hamstrings are engaged as you reach the legs down and toward the floor. Keep the chin up. This will help keep the front of the throat from getting compressed and putting unnecessary pressure on the neck vertebrae.

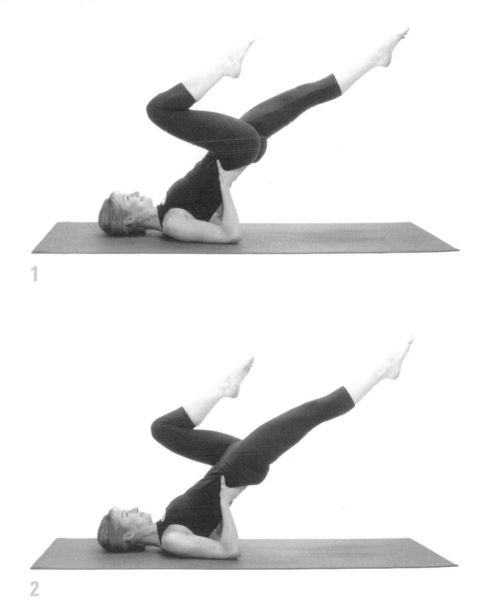

1

2

Boomerang

Begin seated upright with the legs straight and engaged (1). Legs are crossed and externally rotated so that the knees face slightly outward. Torso is in an upright, neutral position, arms are straight, and palms are flat on the floor near the hips. Inhaling, roll to the back of the torso, bringing the legs and pelvis overhead into a modified plow position (2). Keep the arms anchored on the floor. While in this position, quickly change the legs so that the other leg is on top. Exhaling, roll up so that the legs are in the air and crossed, bringing the arms around to the front, reaching them toward the feet so that they are parallel with the legs (3). Inhaling and maintaining this position, bring the arms around behind you and lace the fingers or grasp the hands together (4). Your legs and arms are now on the same diagonal plane. Exhaling, bring the legs to the floor in the same crossed position with control, and flex the torso over the legs. Bring the arms up behind you and parallel to the floor or higher for a shoulder stretch (5). Inhaling, release the hands and sweep the arms out to the sides and forward until they are alongside the head reaching toward the feet (6). Externally rotate the arms immediately as they sweep to the sides so that when they arrive near the head, the palms are facing down. Exhaling, articulate the spine back to the upright, seated position, and bring the arms back to the starting position as well. Repeat. If hamstrings are tight, slightly bend the knees at all times. When moving the arms, anchor the shoulder blades down to avoid hunching the shoulders.

This exercise is contraindicated for those with thoracic osteoporosis or neck issues.

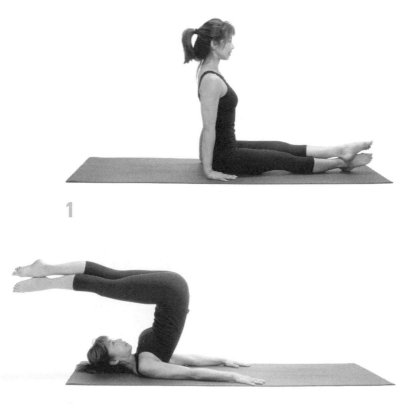

1

2

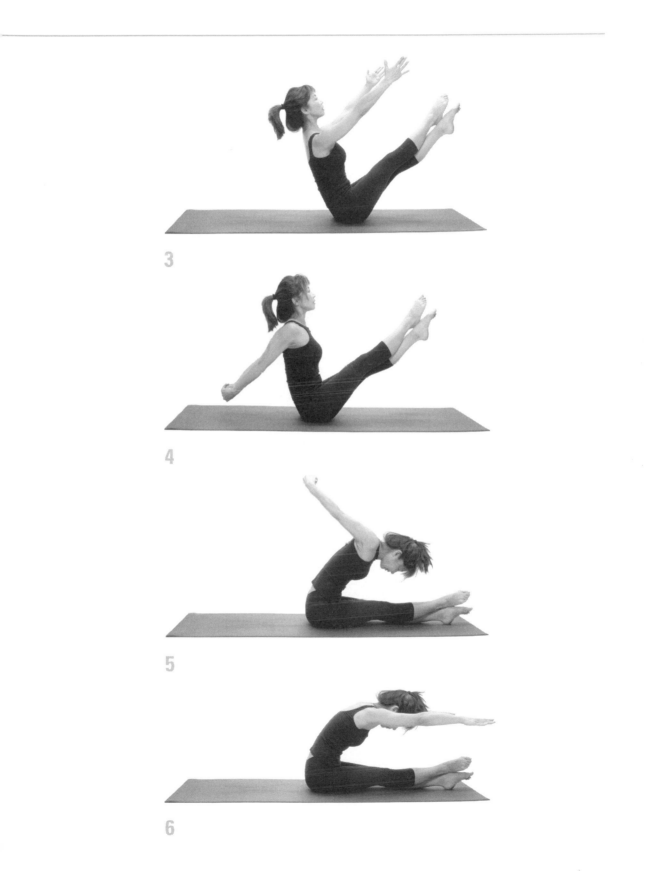

3

4

5

6

Bow (Rocking)

Lying facedown, bend both knees, and grasp the ankles (1). If possible, keep the feet touching. Inhaling, engage the inner unit. Exhaling, simultaneously press the ankles against the hands and bring the upper trunk into extension (2). The thighs may or may not touch the floor. Inhaling, gently rock the upper torso up with the chest lifted. Exhaling, gently rock the upper torso forward onto the chest, keeping the head lifted (3). Be aware not to initiate the rocking movement by jerking the head up and down. This extremely demanding position requires flexibility at the hip flexors, shoulder joints, quadriceps, and spine.

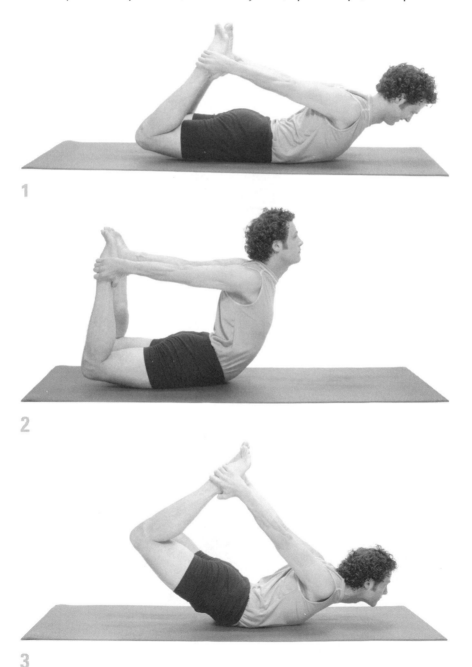

1

2

3

Bridging Scissors

Begin lying on your upper back with both hands under the lower back and propping the hips up in the air, fingers pointing in the direction that is most comfortable for your wrists. The elbows are perpendicular to the wrists with the shoulders rolled underneath you. Both legs are together and reaching toward the ceiling with the toes softly pointed. Inhaling, bring the right leg toward the torso and reach the left leg away from the torso (1). *Continue inhaling* as you switch legs (2). Exhale as you repeat the two scissor movements again. Keep the legs straight to work the flexibility aspect of this exercise, and maintain torso stability throughout the movement phase.

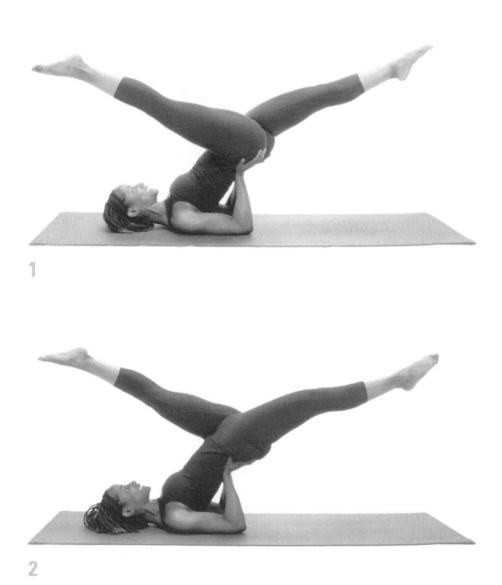

1

2

Cat Twist

Begin on your hands and knees, with the hands placed directly below the shoulders and the knees placed directly below the hips. Head and neck are in line with the neutral spine. Inhaling, turn the left arm inward, pointing the fingers toward the chest with the elbow jutting outward and slightly upward. Exhaling, reach the right arm under the left, rotating the torso (spine) so that you are looking over the top of your left shoulder (1). Allow the spine to rotate and fully arch from tailbone to head at the same time, pulling the chest through. Avoid overturning the neck, and keep the chin aligned with the breastbone. Do not look underneath the top arm. Repeat to the opposite side (2).

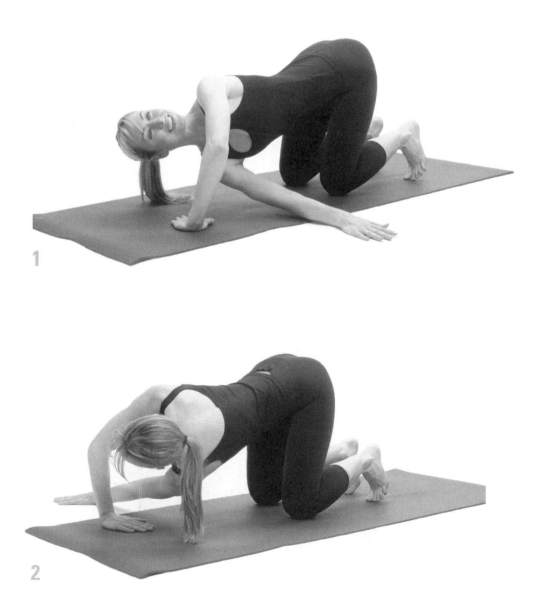

Child's Pose

Facing the floor, begin with your knees bent and buttocks on the heels and the thighs open so that the chest can rest on the legs. Place your arms either behind you, toward your buttocks with the palms up, or place them alongside the head with the palms down. If your buttocks do not rest on your heels, place a cushion or towel that is thick enough so that the buttocks will have something to rest on. Breathe normally in this position.

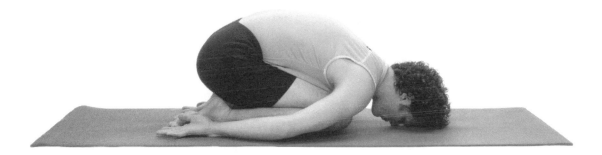

Corkscrew 1

Begin lying on your back with legs to the ceiling, parallel and pressed together, feet softly pointed, arms in a T position. Bend knees if hamstring tightness does not allow you to keep your pelvis neutral. Inhale and tilt the pelvis to one side (1). Exhale and rotate the pelvis away from you (2, lower spine is slightly arching) around to the opposite side (3), then back to the center starting position. Inhale and tip the pelvis to the other side. Exhale and rotate the pelvis away from you, around to the other side and back to the starting position. Repeat alternating sides. The upper torso should remain stabilized, and the opposing back rib cage should not leave the floor.

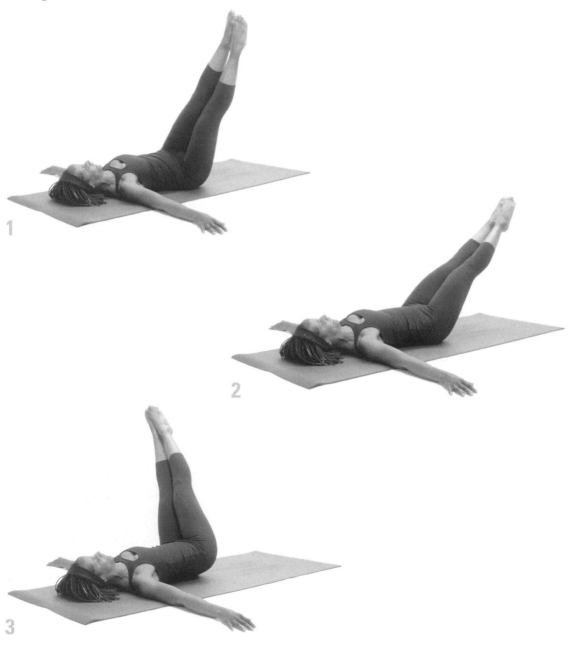

Begin lying on your back with the legs parallel and pressed together in a modified plow position, feet softly pointed (1). Arms are parallel to each other with the palms down toward the floor. Inhaling, roll the spine toward the floor. As you feel the middle back begin to touch, angle the pelvis slightly toward the right (2). Still inhaling, continue moving the spine toward the floor until the pelvis is down (3). As you exhale, rotate the pelvis to sweep the legs around (4), and using the momentum of the legs and contracting the abdominals, continue sweeping the legs and pelvis back to the starting position. Repeat to the other side and alternate sides for 5 complete sets. When you are finished, roll the spine down to the floor using the deep abdominals. This particular exercise requires a shorter inhalation and a longer, controlled exhalation. All movements should be smooth and controlled despite the momentum aspect in this exercise. Anchoring the arms and shoulder blades will assist in stabilizing the upper torso when necessary.

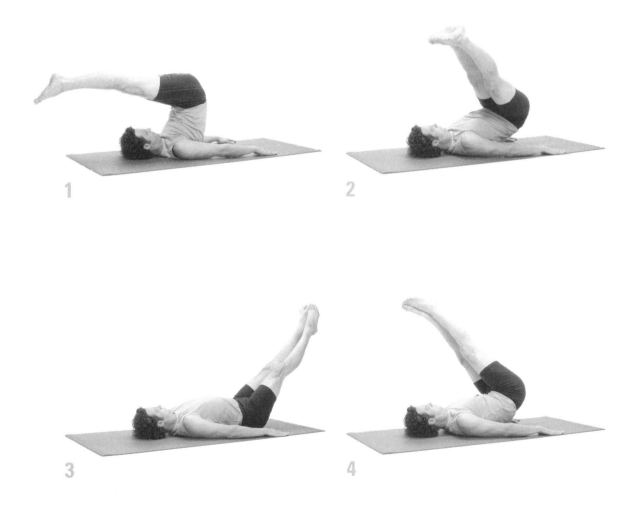

1

2

3

4

Corpse

Begin lying on your back with the arms out and away from the torso and the palms up. Position the legs slightly apart, and let them flop open. Close your eyes and mouth, and relax your jaw. With each progressive breath, allow your face to soften, the corners of your mouth to release, and the space between your eyebrows to open. Feel the tension drain from your body like grains of sands dribbling through an hourglass, slowly and steadily with each subsequent breath. Breathe deeply and completely and let go.

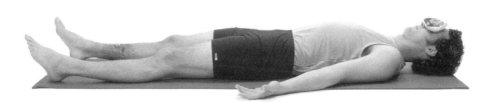

Double-Leg Kick

Lie facedown with the legs together, arms behind you, elbows bent and resting on the floor, with your hands at your lower back (1). Head is turned to one side. Engage the inner unit. As you inhale, bend the knees and pulse the heels toward the buttocks 3 times (2). As you exhale, stretch the arms out behind you with the palms facing inward, stretch the legs long and reach them slightly off the floor, and arch the entire upper torso (3). Keep head and neck in line with the rest of your spine. Inhaling, return to the starting position with your head now turned to the *other* side. Be sure that the elbows relax toward the floor before you repeat the next sequence.

Note: Elbows may or may not be completely resting on the floor. *Do not force elbows to the floor.*

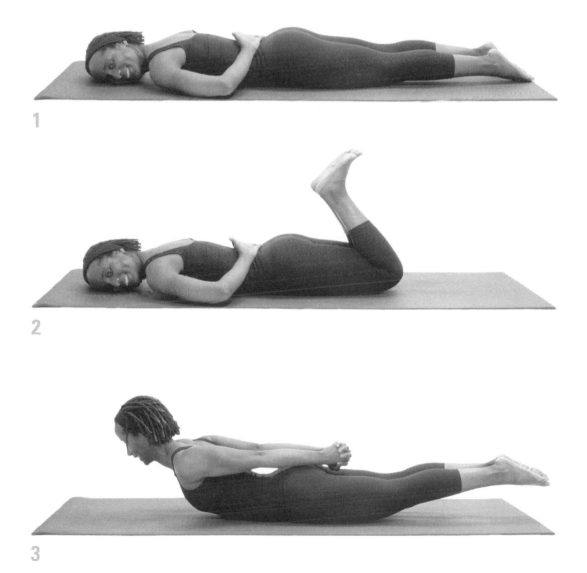

1

2

3

Double-Leg Stretch

Begin lying on your back, knees bent toward the chest, legs together, and feet softly pointed (1). Upper torso is curled forward with the arms reaching toward the ankles on the outside of the legs. Pelvis is in neutral. As you inhale, reach the arms toward the ceiling and back until they are alongside the ears. Simultaneously straighten the legs forward about 45 degrees (2). As you exhale, sweep the arms to the side and forward (3) while bending the knees back to the starting position. Avoid moving the trunk and especially the head and neck when sweeping the arms. Keep the eyes focused forward, and *do not* allow the gaze of the eyes to travel upward, or the head will fall back and strain the neck.

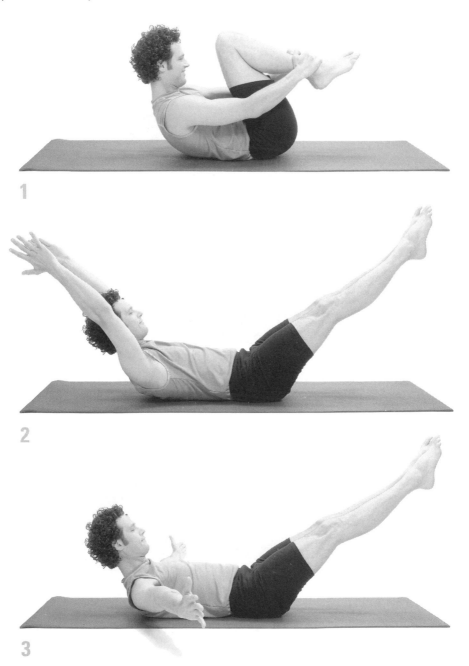

1

2

3

Downward Dog

From a plank position, separate the legs hip-distance apart and press the hips back and up in the air so that the arms, spine, and pelvis form one long diagonal. Press the heels down toward the floor, and fully engage the legs on all sides. Distribute the weight as much as possible onto the legs. Arms are shoulder-distance apart with the neck long. Engage the shoulder blade stabilizers, and lengthen between the armpit and upper side ribs. Be sure that you press the roots of the fingers (located on the palm side of the hand where the large finger knuckles are located) into the floor to avoid bearing all your weight on the base of the palms. Do not allow the ribs to sag toward the floor. The head and neck should be in alignment with the rest of the spine. This is a transitional position between exercises. You may also opt to simply rest in child's pose for a less challenging option.

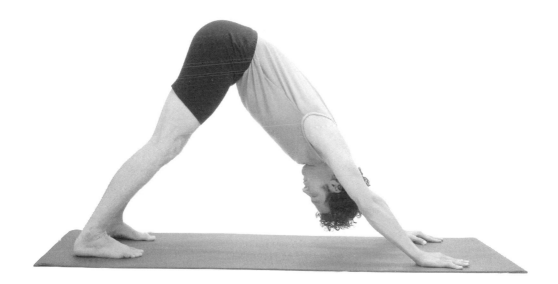

Figure 4 Stretch

Begin lying on your back with your right ankle crossed over the left leg just above the knee. Cross your right outer ankle bone so that it is to the outside of the left thigh with the right knee open to the right. Grasp the left thigh with both hands, and use your right elbow to press the right knee open to increase the stretch. Keep your pelvis as neutral as possible. If your external hip rotators (those are what you are stretching) are too tight and you are unable to grasp your left thigh comfortably, use a strap around that thigh. Be sure to change sides after holding the first side a minimum of 30 seconds.

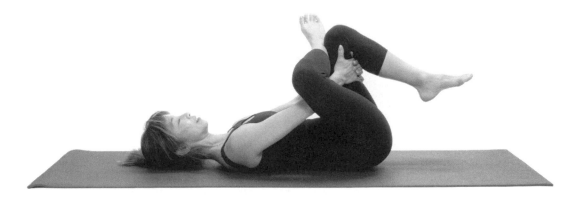

Front Support With Downward Dog and Push-Up

Face the floor in a push-up plank position (1). Legs are straight and together with heels reaching back. Arms are directly below the shoulders to support the weight of the upper torso. Strongly engage the deep abdominals and buttocks to stabilize the pelvis. Keep the legs and torso in one straight line. Inhale. As you exhale, pulse the right leg up behind you twice (2). Inhaling, lower the leg to starting position. Repeat with the other leg. Exhaling, bend the elbows and lower the torso in one long line hovering off of the floor (3). Inhaling, straighten the elbows (4). Exhaling, reach the body back into downward dog position (5). Inhaling, return back to the plank hold position. Repeat for 5 complete cycles (right and left leg pulsing and push-up = 1 set). For a greater challenge, perform additional push-ups.

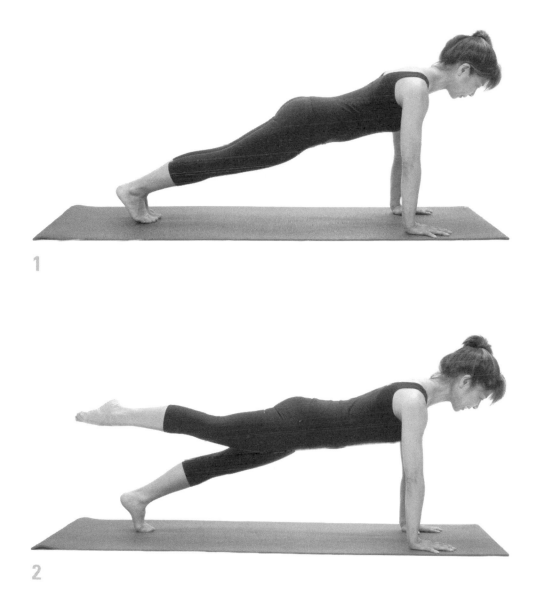

1

2

(continued)

Front Support With Downward Dog and Push-Up

(continued)

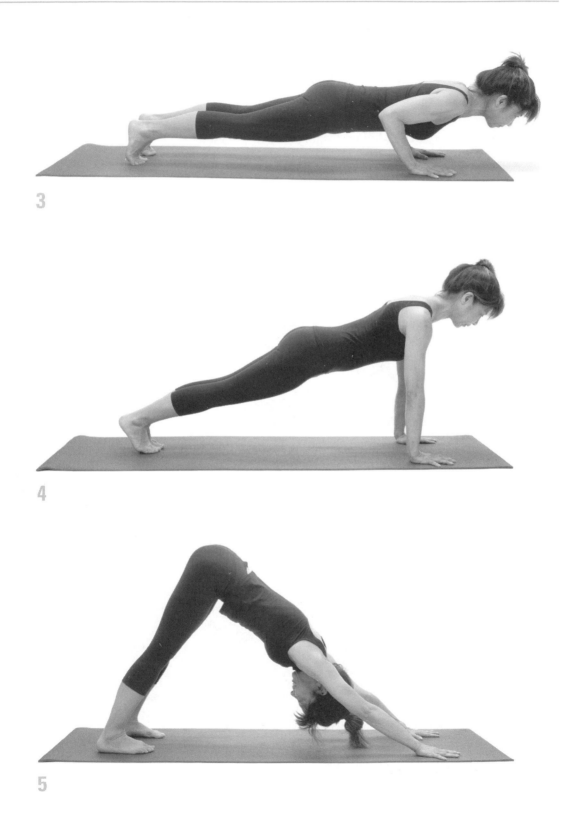

3

4

5

Front Support With Push-Ups

From a hands-and-knees position, bring the feet back with the legs pressed together so that you form a plank shape (1). Hips are in a straight line with your head and neck, shoulders, and knees. Engage the scapulae stabilizers along with the inner unit and lower glutes. Inhale. As you exhale, pulse the leg up behind you twice (2), only as far as possible without disturbing the stability of the pelvis, spine, and shoulders. Inhaling, lower the leg. Repeat again with the other leg. Feel a tension connection from the inner thighs through the pelvic floor to the deep abdominals. Watch that the head and neck do not drop. (I call this "falling into the feedbag.") Add push-ups (3) in at either of these points: between each leg pulse (i.e., pulse right leg twice, perform 1 to 3 push-ups, pulse left leg twice, perform 1 to 3 push-ups) or between sets of leg pulses (i.e., pulse right leg twice, then left leg twice, and perform 1 to 3 push-ups; repeat). All push-ups can be done from knees-on-floor position.

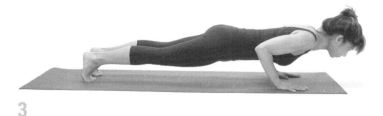

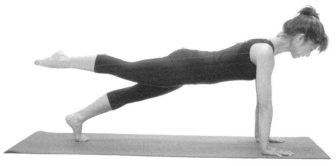

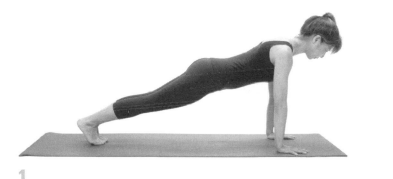

Hamstring and Inner Thigh Stretch With Band

Hamstrings: Begin lying on your back with the left leg bent and left foot flat on the floor. Extend the right leg to the ceiling, the ankle flexed with a strap, both hands grasping the ends of the strap, and the elbows placed on the floor (1). Anchor the pelvis in neutral. Hold the position for 30 to 60 seconds, and repeat with the other leg. *Inner Thigh*: Begin in the same position as for hamstrings, but bring the leg to the outside of the torso avoiding any rocking to the side or hiking up of the pelvis (2). Hold the position for 30 to 60 seconds, and repeat with the other leg.

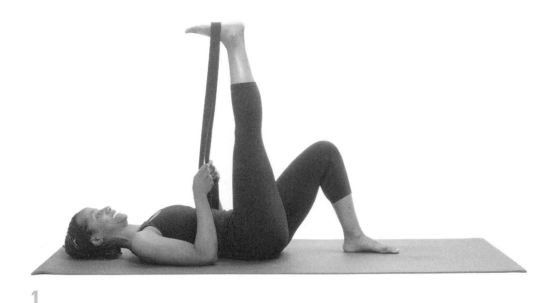

1

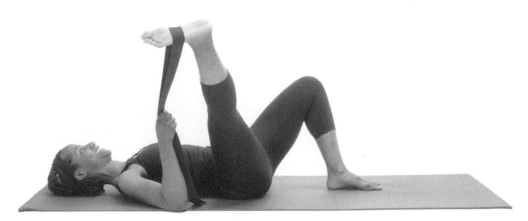

2

Hip Circles

Begin seated upright with the legs off the floor in front of the body, straight and pressed together, and the feet pointed (1). Bend the knees if the hamstrings are too tight. Arms are behind the torso and hands are placed flat on the floor behind the hips. Fingers may be pointed either to the sides or straight back behind the trunk. You may modify the upper torso position by resting on the elbows, but avoid collapsing the chest. Inhaling, tip the hips toward the right, keeping the upper torso still and stable (2). Exhaling, sweep the legs away from you (3) and around to the left (4), returning to the starting position. Inhaling, tip the hips now to the left, keeping the torso quiet. Exhaling, sweep the legs away from you and to the right, returning to the starting position.

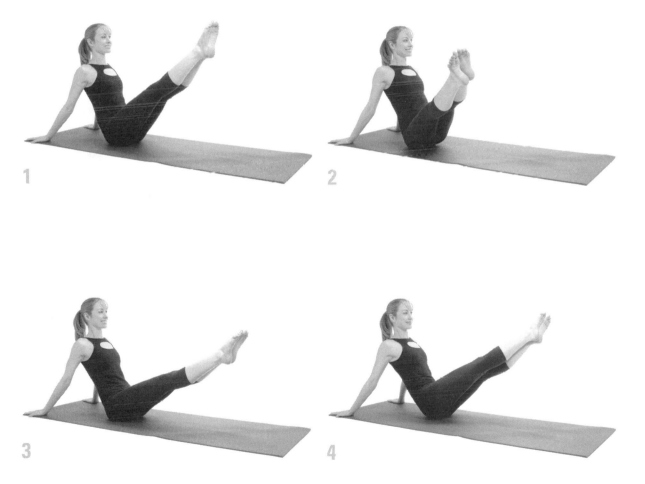

The Hundred

Begin lying on your back with the legs in the air and pressed strongly together. Hips and knees are bent at 90-degree angles, and shins are parallel to the floor. Legs are in a tabletop position (1). Arms are next to your trunk with the palms down. Inhale. As you exhale, bring the upper torso forward, hinging at the T point (located straight back to the spine from the lowest point of the breastbone) and reaching arms toward the feet, hovering parallel to the floor. Simutaneously, legs extend to 45 degrees (2). Pumping the arms up and down, inhale for 5 counts, and exhale for 5 counts. Perform 8 complete cycles. Inhale once again, and as you exhale, engage the abdominals to slowly return the torso and legs back to the starting position. Be sure to keep the pelvis in neutral and the distance from the lower rib to hip bones long. Lengthen across the collar bones as you keep the shoulder blades moving down the back. Keep your eyes focused forward toward the inner thighs.

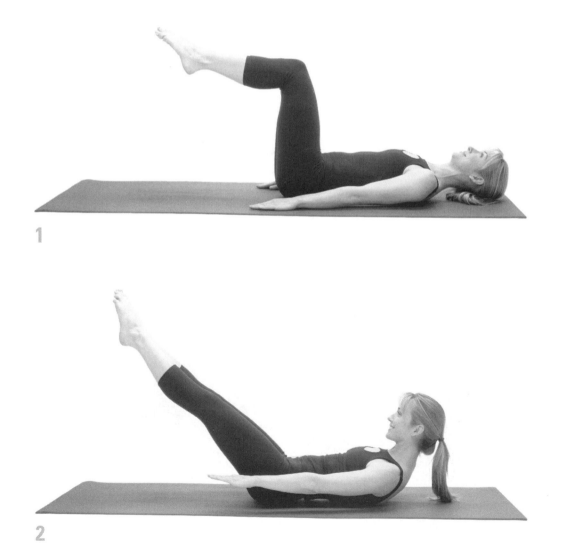

1

2

Jackknife

Lying on your back with the legs together, reach the legs straight up for the ceiling, forming a 90-degree angle at the hip joint (1). If your hamstrings are restricting this position, slightly bend the knees. Strongly use the inner thigh muscles to keep the legs together throughout this exercise. Arms are alongside the torso, palms facing down. Inhaling, deeply engage the abdominals to tilt the pelvis back. Do not initiate movement from the legs; they are just along for the ride. Exhaling, engage the deep abdominals to reach the legs overhead to a plow position (2) and then using the hamstrings and glutes, immediately reach the legs straight up to a shoulder stand (3). Strongly recruit the leg muscles to achieve this position. Inhaling, fold at the hip joint back to about 45 degrees (4). Exhaling, control the articulation of the spine back down to the starting position while reaching the legs strongly in the opposite direction. Avoid dropping the legs toward the chest, and keep the hip joint open.

This exercise is contraindicated for those with neck problems, as well as those with thoracic osteoporosis.

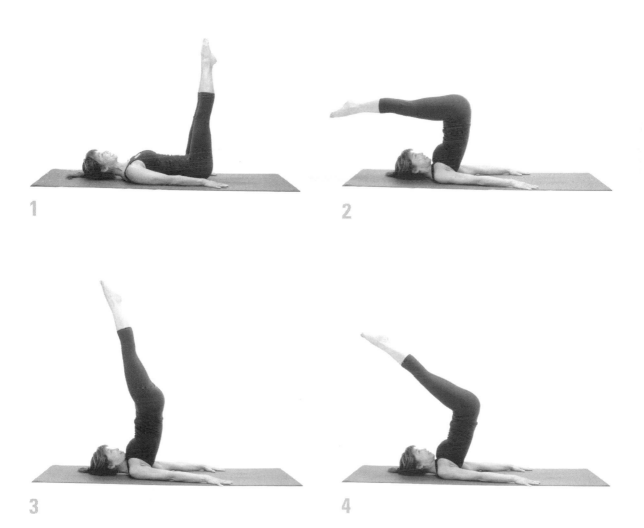

1

2

3

4

Lunge (Standing)

Stand with one foot placed forward to assume a lunging position. The back leg is straight with the heel off the floor. The front leg is bent at the knee approximately 90 degrees. Square the hips and shoulders, placing the shoulder girdle directly above the pelvic girdle (avoid leaning forward or back). The pelvis is level and not rotated. Bring the arms upward alongside the ears with the palms facing in. Exhaling, bend the front knee a bit deeper and reach the back leg slightly straighter. Feel a stretch in the front of the hip and thigh of the back leg (hip flexor and upper quadriceps). Keep the tailbone drawn in without overgripping the buttocks. Reach both arms up with the shoulder blades anchoring down the back. Hold for 30 to 60 seconds. Repeat to the other side.

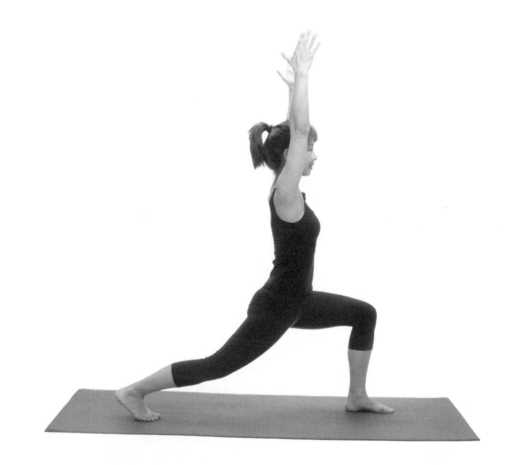

Mermaid

Begin seated sideways with knees slightly bent and legs stacked (1). Top foot is slightly in front of the bottom one. Bottom hand is resting on the floor slightly wider than the shoulder. Top arm is resting on the side of the top leg. Inhaling, straighten legs, bringing the torso over the supporting arm. Legs are stacked and parallel, the outside edge of the bottom foot firmly anchored into the floor (2). Both ankles are flexed with the top arm lightly resting on the side of the top leg. Deeply engage the abdominals, lower glutes, inner thighs, and hamstrings. Exhaling, side bend the torso and bring the hips toward the floor, strongly stretching the underside of the torso and hip area (3). Top arm slides slightly toward the knee and the face turns to look toward the feet. Keep the neck long. Inhaling, return to neutral diagonal position and reach top arm alongside the ear, keeping the shoulder blade anchored down the back as the face turns to look straight down at the floor slightly beyond the supporting hand (4). Exhaling and bending knees, return with control to the starting position. Feel the front body press into the back body to help keep your balance. Strongly engage the shoulder blade stabilizers, especially of the supporting arm, to avoid collapsing on that side. Also, engage all four sides of the legs to help keep your balance as well. Repeat to the other side after 4 to 6 reps.

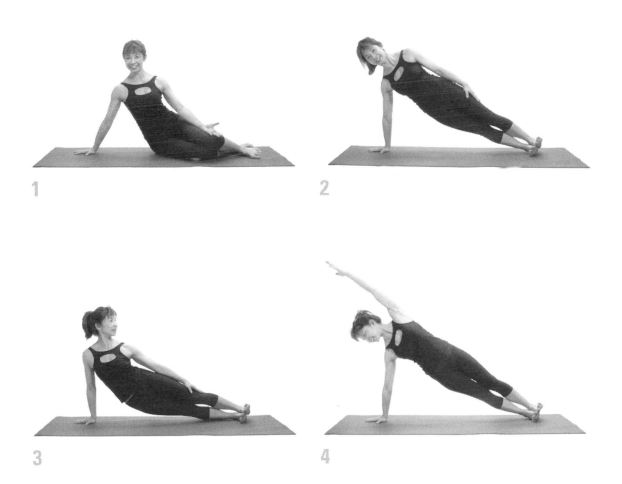

1

2

3

4

Neck Pull

Begin lying on your back, with fingers interlaced and placed behind the neck, the outside edge of the pinky finger at the base of the skull (1). Elbows are lifted slightly off of the floor, pointing outward, and legs are straight and pressed together with the ankles flexed. As you inhale, bring the head, neck, and shoulders forward off the floor, keeping the elbows in the same position (2). Avoid pushing the neck or head forward! As you exhale, continue flexing the entire torso forward, articulating through each vertebra of the spine until you cannot curl forward any further (3). Inhaling, bring the torso upright (4). Keep the length through the spine as much as possible. Exhaling, begin to tilt the pelvis back (5) but keep the upper torso lifted, and continue to exhale and articulate the spine back to the starting position. Maintain the position of the arms when moving up or down from the floor, and maintain a lengthened sensation throughout the spine even when you are flexing the torso. To decrease difficulty, legs may be slightly apart with ankles flexed or arms may be crossed in front of the chest.

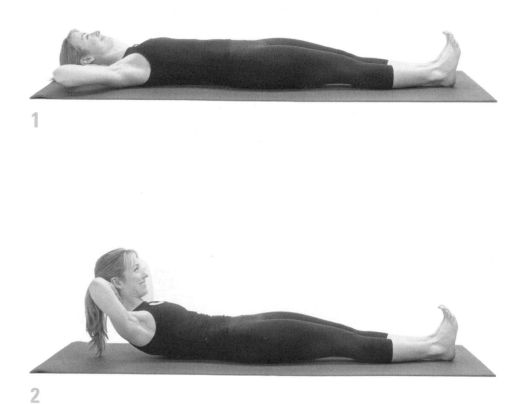

1

2

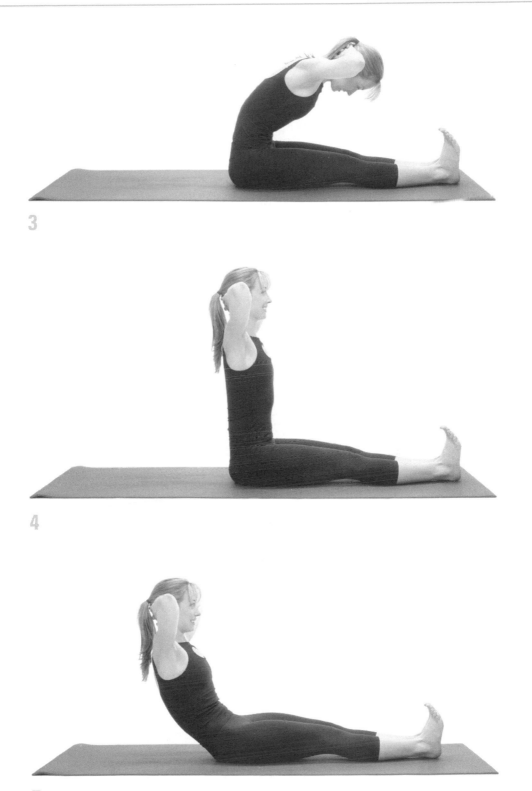

3

4

5

Oblique Rotation With Longer Breaths

Begin lying on your back with fingers interlaced behind the neck and elbows pointing outward. Right knee is bent toward you; the left leg is stretched out straight ahead (1). Inhaling, rotate the torso while bringing the left shoulder toward the right bent knee (2), and *continue inhaling* as you rotate the right shoulder to the left bent knee. Exhaling, again rotate the right shoulder to the left bent knee. Continue exhaling as you rotate the right shoulder to the left bent knee. Maintain wide elbows so that the rotation is isolated in the trunk and not falsified with simply driving the elbow across the face. The pelvis is anchored in neutral. Move slowly and deliberately to correctly isolate the rotational aspect in the rib cage. Pay attention to keeping the upper torso flexed forward so that you avoid simply rolling side to side and not working to full capacity.

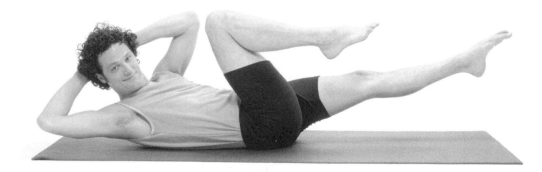

1

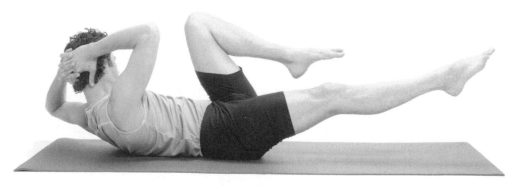

2

Oblique Scissors

Begin lying on your back with fingers interlaced behind the neck and elbows pointing outward. Both legs are straight, the right leg toward you and the left leg stretched out straight ahead (split position). Inhaling, rotate the torso, bringing the left shoulder toward the right knee (1). *Continue inhaling* as you rotate the right shoulder to the left knee (2). Exhaling, again rotate the left shoulder to the right knee. *Continue exhaling* as you rotate the right shoulder to the left knee. Legs remain straight at all times. Maintain the elbows wide so that the rotation is isolated in the trunk and not falsified with simply driving the elbow across the face. The pelvis is anchored in neutral. Keep the upper torso flexed forward to avoid simply rolling side to side and not working to full capacity.

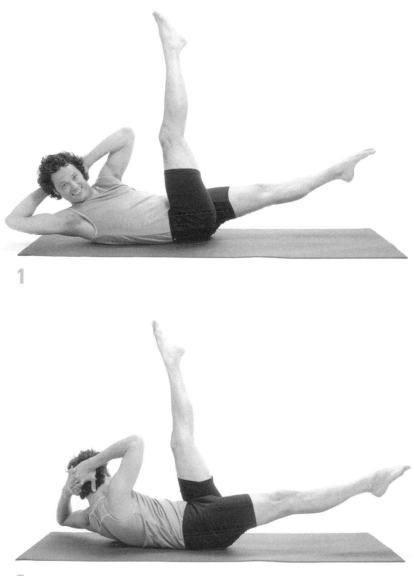

1

2

Open-Leg Rocker

Begin balanced just in back of the tailbone, with the legs straight, shoulder-distance apart, and the hands grasping the top of the ankles (1). Keep the arms straight, toes softly pointed, and spine slightly flexed. Inhale. As you exhale, engage the abdominals to roll back to just the upper back (2). Continue exhaling to return to the starting position. It is essential to keep the arms and legs straight throughout the entire movement phase. The spine is slightly flexed to ensure even rolling. Use the abdominals (through the breath) as the impetus for rolling back as well as to brake the upward movement to stop in the starting position. Never roll onto the neck.

This exercise is contraindicated for those with neck problems and those with thoracic osteoporosis.

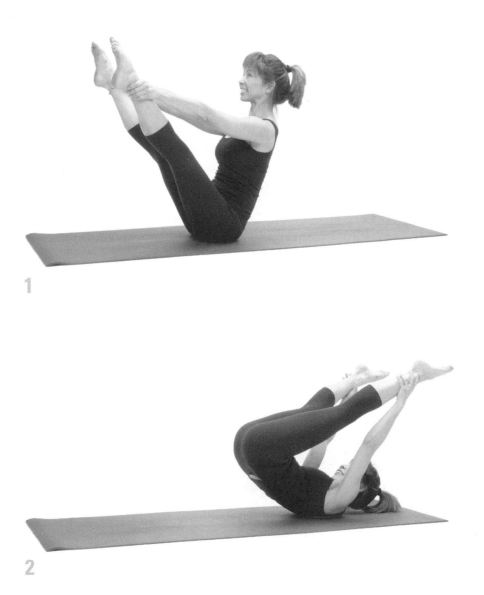

1

2

Open and Close Leg Rocker

Begin balanced just in back of the tailbone with legs straight, shoulder-distance apart, and hands grasping the top of the ankles (1). Arms are straight as well, toes softly pointed, spine very slightly flexed, chest lifted. Inhale. As you exhale, roll back to just the upper back (2) while bringing the legs together using the inner thighs (3). Continue to exhale as you return to the starting position while keeping the legs together (4). Inhale as you open the legs. Exhaling, roll back again, closing the legs together. Continue exhaling to rock back up. Repeat 5 times in this direction. From the previous position (which should end upright with the legs together), inhale again. Exhaling, roll back onto the upper back as you open the legs to a V position, then continue to exhale as you roll back up to the starting position, keeping the legs apart.

This exercise is contraindicated for those with neck issues as well as those with thoracic osteoporosis.

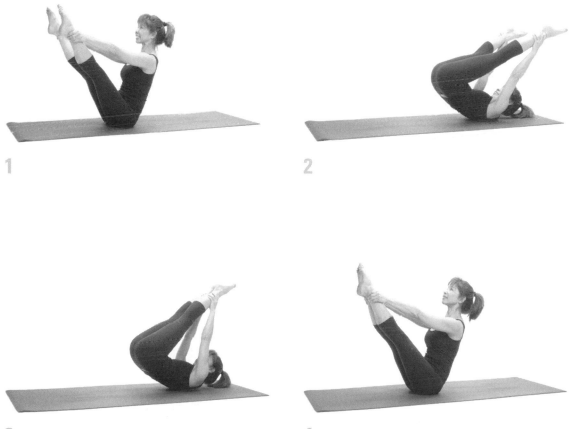

1

2

3

4

Pelvic Peel With Leg Abduction and Adduction

Begin lying on your back with feet flat on the floor (1). Knees are bent, heels are in line with the sit bones, and arms are next to your trunk with the palms down. Inhale. Exhaling, slowly peel spine away from the floor, articulating through each vertebra until the hips are in a straight diagonal line with the shoulders and knees (2). Inhaling, slowly straighten the right knee, keeping the thighs parallel (3). Exhaling, slowly move the leg slightly to the outside of the torso line (abduction), maintaining the stability of the neutral pelvis (4). Do not allow the left knee to wander off to the side. Do not overarch the spine when carrying the leg into abduction. Inhaling, bring the right leg back to parallel with the left thigh. Exhaling, bend the knee and replace the foot on the floor. Inhaling, straighten the left knee, keeping stable. Exhaling, carry the left leg slightly to the side. Inhaling, return the left leg back to the parallel position. Exhaling, bend the left knee and replace the foot on the floor. Inhale. Exhaling, articulate the spine back down to the supine starting position. On the way down, draw the abdominals away from the knees. Use your inner thighs to draw the tailbone away from you when rolling down to feel a tractioning length through the spine. Avoid oversqueezing the buttocks. Distribute your workload so that you feel the front of the body just as much as the back of the body.

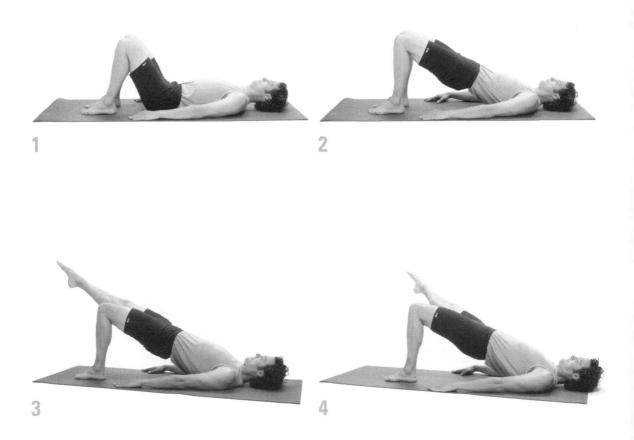

1

2

3

4

Begin lying on your back with knees bent, heels in line with sitting bones (1). Inhale. Exhaling, slowly peel the spine away from the floor starting at the tailbone (2). Articulate through each vertebra until your hips are in a straight diagonal line with the shoulders and knees (3). Inhale. Exhaling, begin returning to the starting position from the upper back, articulating through each vertebra using the inner thighs, and drawing the tailbone away from you. Repeat twice. Then, for the next 2 reps, repeat as described but this time, allow the hips to press beyond neutral to open the front of the hip joints, stretching the hip flexors. When articulating, work to synchronize the spinal movement to the breath. Do not allow the knees to splay open at any time.

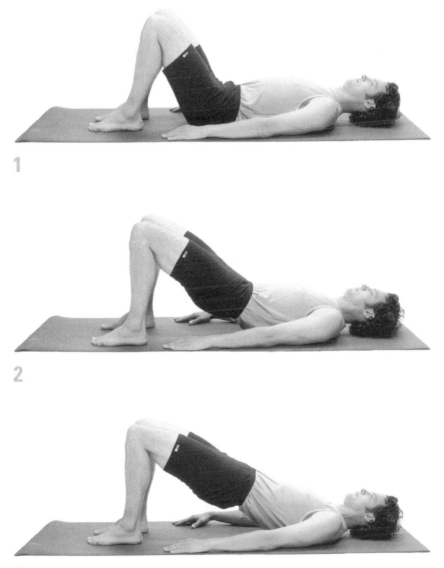

1

2

3

Quad Release

Begin seated upright in a side sitting position. Lean to one side, resting on that elbow and forearm. Bottom knee is bent slightly in front of you, and top leg is bent at the knee with the thigh in line with the torso. Avoid collapsing the trunk sideways. Grasp the top ankle, and engage the abdominals to stabilize the pelvis. Gently press the ankle into the hand and feel a stretch across the length of the front of the thigh (quadriceps). If the thigh is extremely tight and causes you to tilt your pelvis forward (anterior tilt), use a strength band around the ankle to add some length to the arm. Hold for 30 to 60 seconds, then change sides.

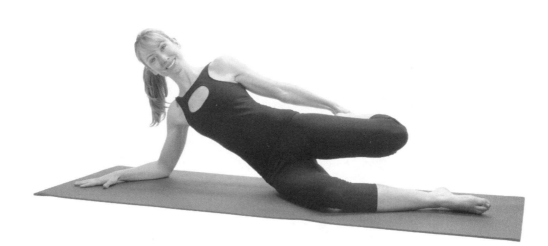

Rollover

Begin lying on your back with your arms at your sides, palms down, and legs together and reaching to the ceiling with the feet softly pointed (1). If the hamstrings are tight, you may slightly bend the knees. Inhale. As you exhale, begin rolling the pelvis back using the abdominals as you curl the spine (tail end) toward you. Your legs will begin to reach toward your head into a modified plow position (2). Inhale as you open the legs shoulder-distance apart and flex the ankles (3). As you exhale, begin articulating the spine sequentially one vertebra at a time back toward the floor with control (4). Return to the starting position. Inhale as you bring the legs together using the inner thighs, and point the feet. Exhale, and repeat the movements. Repeat 5 times, then repeat 5 more times initiating the rollover with the legs apart. Be sure to "ride the wave of the breath" so that all movements are smooth and controlled. If the hamstrings are tight, be sure to bend the knees.

This exercise is contraindicated for those individuals with thoracic osteoporosis and preexisting neck problems.

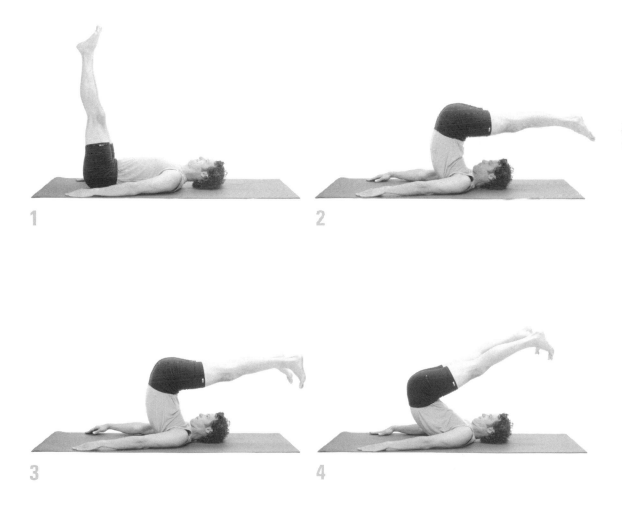

1

2

3

4

Roll-Up (Advanced)

Begin lying on your back with legs apart and ankles flexed (1). Arms are reaching long overhead outside of the ears, off of the floor, a bit wider than the shoulders with the palms facing one another. Spine is in neutral, and the inner unit is fired. Inhaling, bring the arms to a perpendicular position straight above the shoulders (2). Bring the head and neck up to look through the frame formed by the arms toward your feet. Exhaling and *keeping the arms next to the ears,* flex the upper torso and sequentially articulate the spine until the torso is reaching toward the feet and the arms are parallel to the floor above the legs (3). Keep the movement sequence fluid. Inhale in this position. Exhaling, articulate the spine back to the starting position while keeping the arms outside of the ears as much as possible without elevating the shoulders.

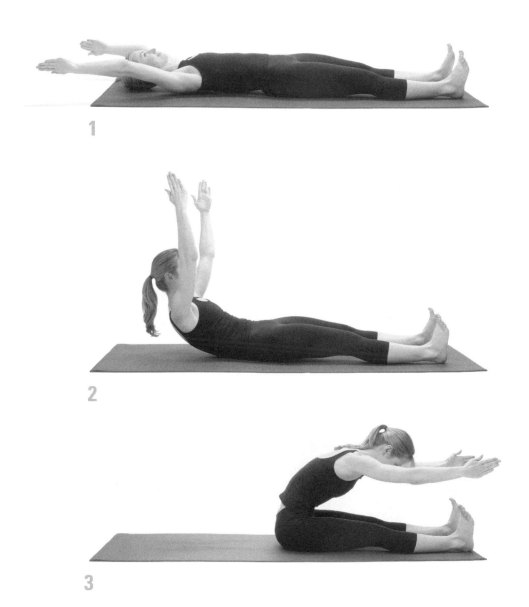

1

2

3

Roll-Up With Twisting Lat Pull

Begin lying on your back with legs parallel and slightly apart, ankles flexed (1). Arms are slightly wider than shoulder-width apart, reaching overhead outside of the ears, off of the floor, and hands grasp a strength band. The band has enough tension to feel the shoulder blade stabilizers working. Inhaling and keeping the band taut, bring the arms to a perpendicular position straight above the shoulders. Bring the head and neck up to look through the frame formed by the arms toward the feet. Lower the arms over the legs, and exhaling, flex the upper torso and roll up until the torso is reaching toward the feet with the arms parallel to the floor above the legs (2). Inhaling, bring the spine upright (3). Exhaling, rotate the torso to the left (the twist) with the arms stretching the band across the upper chest (4). Inhaling, rotate the torso back to center, bringing the arms back overhead. Repeat to the right side. Inhaling, bring the torso to the forward flexed position with arms parallel to the floor and back of the neck long. Exhaling, return to the starting position. Breath may be reversed on the twist for deeper rotation of the spine.

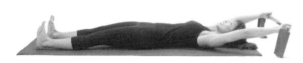

1

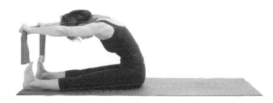

2

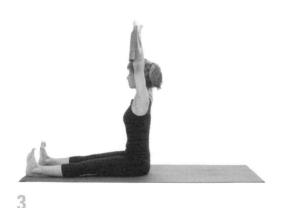

3

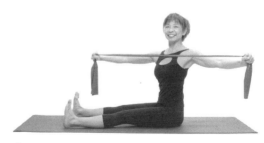

4

Saw With Back Extension

Begin seated upright with your pelvis in neutral position, legs apart slightly wider than shoulder distance, and ankles flexed (1). Leg muscles are fully engaged at all times. Arms are out to the sides, at shoulder height. Engage the inner unit. Inhaling, rotate the torso to the left (2). Keep the pelvis stable. Exhaling, flex the torso forward, reaching the right hand toward the left foot (3). Look toward the back arm if possible; if the neck feels strained, look toward the front hand. Inhale as you bring the torso back up, still rotated to the left and arch back, lifting the chest (spine extension), leaning slightly back on the left hand (4). Feel a tension connection from the lower ribs to the sacral base to support the lumbar spine. As you exhale, return the torso back upright to the starting position. Repeat to the other side.

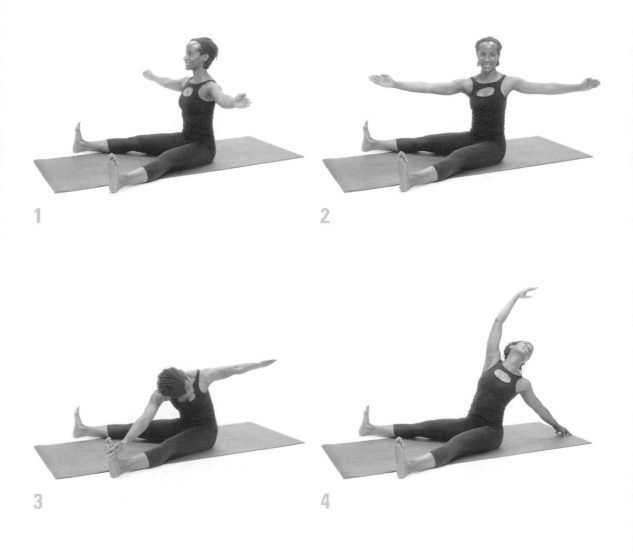

1

2

3

4

Begin lying on your back, pelvis neutral. Bring one leg toward the torso with the hands grasping the back of the leg (1). Keep the leg straight! Reach the other leg long and away, bringing it to about a 45-degree angle or lower if you have no back strain. Fully engage muscles of both legs. As you inhale, perform a scissor action with the legs, switching their position as well as hand hold (2). As you exhale, scissor the legs while you switch again. Pelvis must remain in neutral position! When switching legs, keep them fairly close together. You can further challenge respiratory strength by inhaling for two changes and exhaling for two changes.

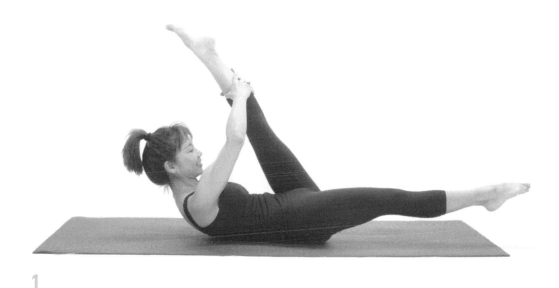

1

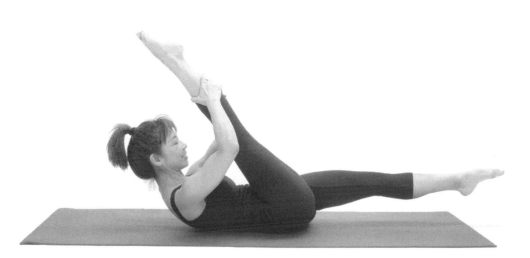

2

Seal (Advanced)

Seated upright, bend knees, and fold the legs toward the torso with the knees opened to the sides. Reach both arms to the inside of the legs and grasp the outside of each ankle with the same-side hand (1). Bring the feet up so that they are approximately in front of the navel. Slightly flex the spine using the abdominals without collapsing the chest so that you can balance just behind the tailbone and in front of the sit bones. Inhaling, clap the feet together twice. Exhaling, roll back (2) and clap the feet together twice while pausing in the inverted position. Note the foot position in the last photo (3). Roll from the tailbone to the top of the upper back only, never onto the neck. Continue to exhale as you roll back up to the starting position. Keep the spine curved at all times, and use the abdominals to create the movement back as well as to brake the movement when returning upright. Engage the pelvic floor at all times to assist in balance and control.

This exercise is contraindicated for those participants with thoracic osteoporosis or pre-existing neck issues.

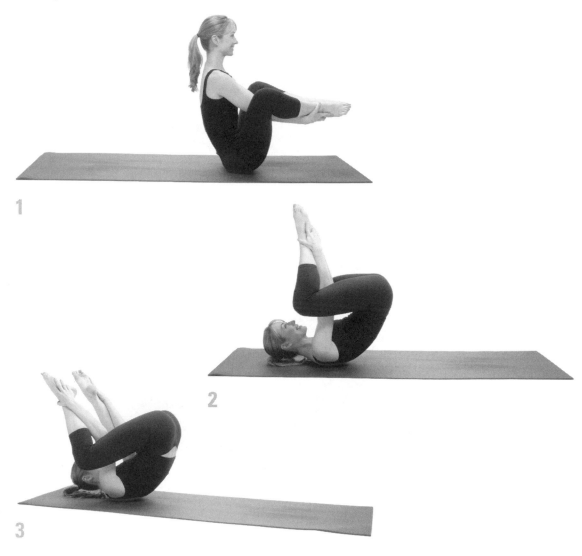

1

2

3

Seated Hip Stretch

Seated upright, cross one leg over the other in a figure 4 position. Top leg is bent at the knee, with the outside ankle bone just above the opposite knee and outside the thigh. The top leg's knee will be to the outside of torso. Ankle is flexed. Place your hands slightly behind the torso, and lean back with a neutral spine and pelvis. Chest stays lifted. Draw the bottom leg up toward you, keeping the top leg placed so that the knee is kept to the outside. You will begin to feel a stretch in the outside hip area of the top leg. Bring the leg in as close as possible while maintaining a neutral pelvis. Don't allow the spine to collapse back. If you have low-back problems, you may recline and opt for the figure 4 stretch on page 178.

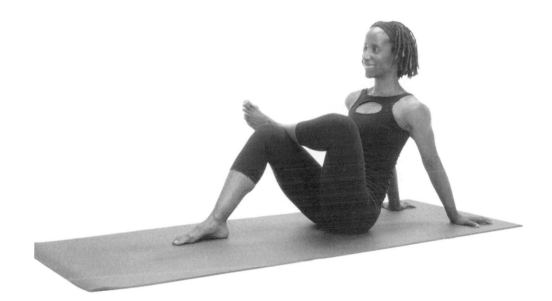

Side Bend

Begin seated sideways, the top leg bent at the knee and the sole of that foot flat on the floor (1). The bottom leg is also bent at the knee with the side of the leg resting on the floor. Hand of the bottom arm is placed flat on the floor just slightly wider than the shoulder, fingers pointing away from the torso. Top arm is resting on the top knee with the palm up. Inhaling, straighten the legs and lift the hips up in the air (2). Press the legs together with the inner thigh muscles. Top arm sweeps in a large arc over the head. The shoulder of the weight-bearing arm must be strongly stabilized using the scapular stabilizers. Reach the hips upward so that the torso, legs, and arm assume the shape of a large crescent. Use the muscles in the hip on the side that is toward the floor to assist in elevating the height of the hips, and engage the leg muscles. Exhaling, return the legs, arm, and torso back to the starting position with control.

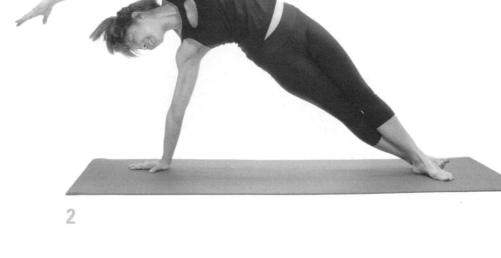

1

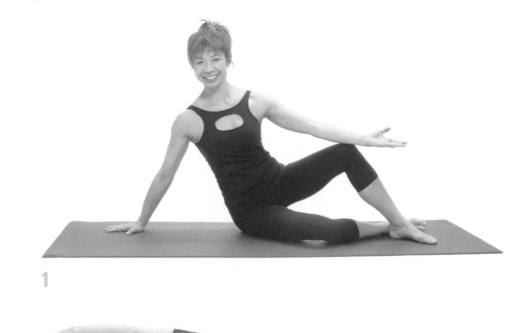

2

Side Kick (Kneeling)

Begin in a kneeling position. Place your right hand on the floor so that it is perpendicular to the right shoulder joint. At the same time bring your left leg up in the same straight line as your torso, parallel to the floor with the kneecap pointing straight ahead of you, foot pointed (1). Keep the bottom right shin at a slight angle, not straight back, to have good balance. The left hand is placed behind the head with the elbow pointing up to the ceiling. Strongly engage the T point (located straight back to the spine from the lowest point of the breastbone) to avoid flaring your rib cage. Inhaling, bring the top leg forward, flexing at the hip and ankle, and pulse the leg twice, sniffing the breath in with the pulse (2). Exhaling, point the foot and carry the leg back behind you, only as far as you can maintain your neutral pelvis and stable torso (3). Keep the leg parallel to the floor, and avoid letting it drift up or down in height. Feel leg movement, not pelvic movement. Repeat.

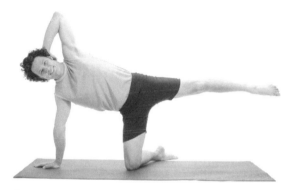

1

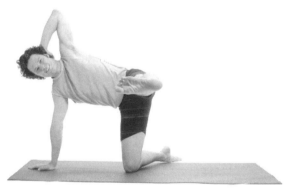

2

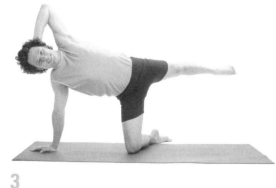

3

Side Kick With Bent Elbows

Begin lying on your side with both legs straight and angled about 20 degrees in front of you at the hip. The ankle of bottom leg is flexed, and the foot of top leg is pointed. Both arms are bent at the elbow and placed behind the head. The entire underside of your torso is off of the floor and in a straight diagonal line with the hips. Strongly engage the T point (located straight back to the spine from the lowest point of the breastbone) to avoid flaring your rib cage. Inhaling, bring the top leg parallel to the floor, reaching long out of the hips and flexing the ankle (1). Exhaling, maintain this position with the deep abdominals and back muscles. Press the outside of the bottom leg into the floor to keep stable. Inhaling, bring the top leg forward, flexing at the hip and ankle, and pulse the leg twice, sniffing the breath in (2). Exhaling, point the foot and carry the leg back behind you, only as far as you can maintain your neutral pelvis (3). Repeat 6 to 8 times, then repeat to the other side.

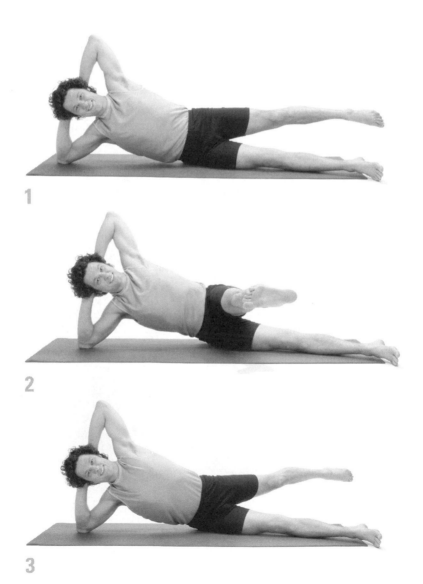

1

2

3

Single-Leg Kick (Advanced)

Begin lying on your front, propped up on your elbows with the hands made into fists (1). Elbows are directly below the shoulders, forearms angled in so that fists are together. Legs are extended straight behind you very close together, slightly hovering off of the floor. Strongly engage the inner unit, and keep the pubic bone anchored on the mat. As you inhale, bend one knee with the ankle flexed and pulse twice gently toward the buttock (2). As you exhale, slowly extend the leg and return it to the starting position, off of the floor (3). Repeat with the other leg. Resist the movement of straightening the knee with your hamstrings. You may place the head down on the hands if the lower back feels compressed, or you may perform the previous version with the legs resting on the floor. Be aware of collapsing in the head and neck area, and avoid it by pressing the forearms firmly into the floor.

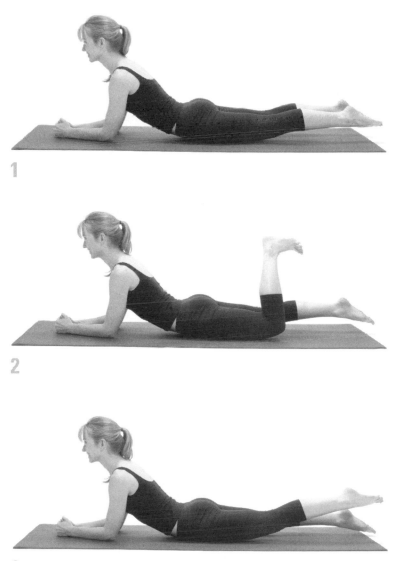

1

2

3

Single-Leg Stretch

Begin lying on your back with the pelvis in neutral and the upper torso flexed forward. Bring one knee toward the chest with the outside hand placed at the ankle and the inside hand placed at the same knee (1). Reach the other leg long into the distance, bringing it to about a 45-degree angle or lower if you have no back strain. Inhale as you switch legs, changing hand position as well (2). Exhale as you switch leg and hand position again. Be sure to keep the elbows wide with the shoulders down. It is hand over hand to change hand position with the leg switch. Repeat, maintaining your neutral pelvis. You can further challenge respiratory strength by inhaling for two changes and exhaling for two changes.

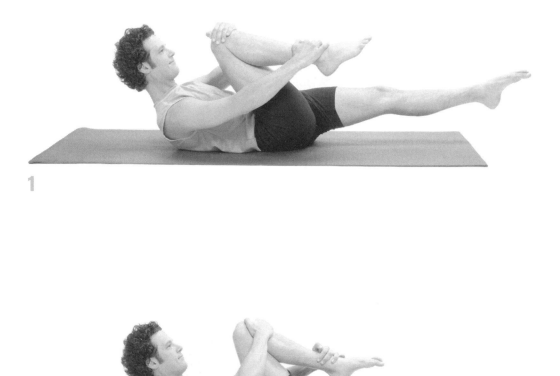

1

2

Spine Spiral With Arms Up

Begin seated upright with legs parallel, stretched straight in front of you, and pressed together (1). Arms are reaching up alongside the head, palms facing in. Feet are flexed at the ankle, and legs are engaged. Torso is in an upright, neutral position. Inhaling, rotate the upper torso to the right with a double pulse, keeping both arms up (2). Exhaling, rotate the torso back to starting position, keeping the arms in the same position. Repeat to the other side (3). Begin your rotation from the lower ribs. Imagine you are spiraling upward as you rotate the torso, and maintain the uplifted spine when rotating back to starting position. Arms stay in the elevated position throughout the exercise. The pelvis should not rock or shift. Breath can be reversed.

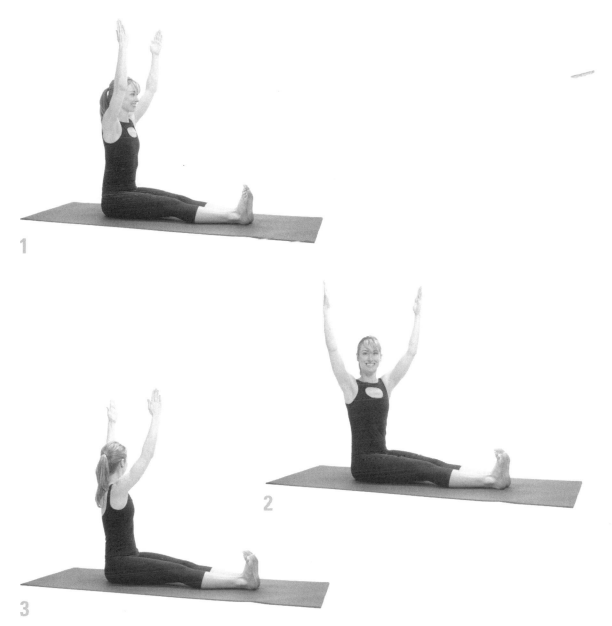

Spine Stretch With Extension

Begin sitting upright with the legs stretched in front of you straight and opened to approximately 90 degrees with the ankles flexed (1). Bend the knees if hamstring shortness prevents an upright, neutral pelvis. Stretch the arms in front of you, parallel to the floor, at shoulder height with the palms down. Inhale to prepare and lengthen the spine. As you exhale, flex the spine forward until the fingertips touch the floor (2). Inhale *in this position.* Exhaling, slide the fingers forward, increasing the flexion of the spine. Avoid collapsing in the chest and shoulders. Inhale in the flexed spine position. As you exhale, return the spine, vertebra by vertebra, to the starting position (1). Inhale as you place the hands on the floor behind the hips (3) and arch the upper torso slightly back (spinal extension). Exhale as you return to the starting position.

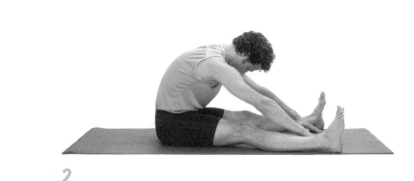

1

2

3

Swan (Rocking)

Lie on your front, elbows bent, hands placed flat near the shoulders, elbows pointing towards the legs (1). Legs are reaching behind you, straight, slightly turned out, approximately 6 to 8 inches (15 to 20 centimeters) apart. Inhale and bring the upper trunk into extension via the back muscles with some assistance from the arms (2). Be sure that the legs are engaged and reaching long out of the hips. Exhaling, "dive" the torso toward the floor as the arms immediately reach forward (3). Utilize the momentum to assist the "diving" movement as well as the strength of the legs reaching out and upward into extension. Inhaling, bring the upper trunk into extension with the arms now assisting the upward movement (4). The inhalation at this point will assist in bringing the torso upward. Exhaling, again utilize the momentum of the upper torso rocking. The energy and "distribution" of work should reach through the entire body at all times. This exercise is quite dynamic and uses a lot of momentum. Be sure to keep the legs and inner unit fully engaged!

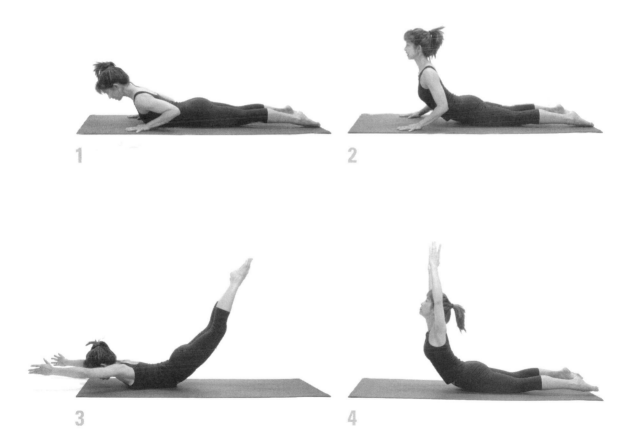

1

2

3

4

Swimming

Begin lying on your front with the arms and legs reaching in opposite directions. Keep the legs parallel, heels in line with the sitting bones. The face and chest are hovering off the floor, with the head and neck aligned with the rest of the spine. Inhaling, move the opposing arm and leg slightly higher away from the floor in a swimming motion for four movements (1). Exhaling, repeat again, moving the opposing arm and leg for four movements (2). Be sure to reach the arm and leg off the floor only as far as you do not disturb the stability of your pelvis and shoulder girdle.

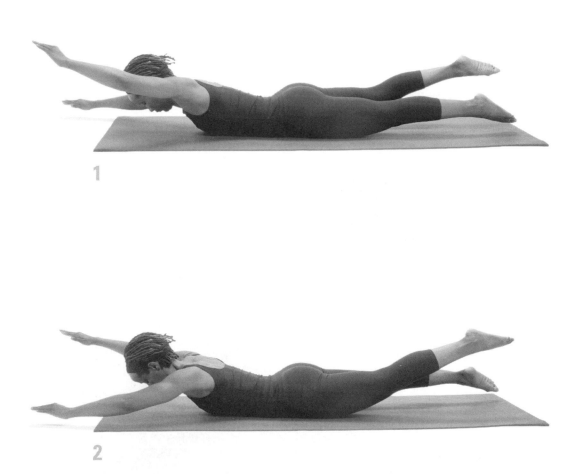

1

2

Begin seated upright and balanced just slightly behind the tailbone, with the legs up in front of you in the air, pressed together and parallel, feet pointed (1). Arms are reaching toward the feet on the same diagonal line as the legs. Torso is lifted and erect. Inhaling, sequentially articulate the spine back toward the floor with control as you simultaneously lower the legs (2). The arms come along for the ride and end up placed alongside the ears (3). Exhaling, sequentially articulate the spine back up to the starting position while simultaneously bringing the legs up from the floor as the arms come forward toward the legs with control. Finish in the starting position. Perform the entire sequence smoothly and in a controlled manner. It is very easy to make a chopping motion with the arms and rely solely on the hip flexors to return to the starting position. Resist this type of motion. Work to bring the legs and torso up and down in a symmetrical manner.

As a variation, sweep the arms to the sides on the way up or down as in the double-leg stretch.

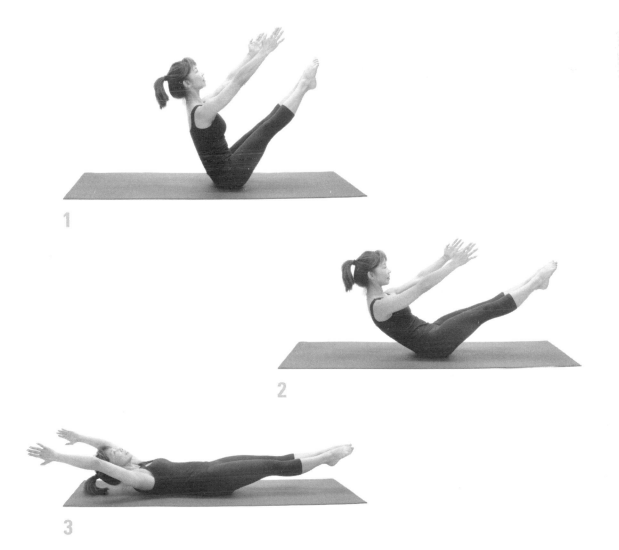

1

2

3

Twist

Begin seated sideways with the top leg bent at the knee and the sole of that foot flat on the floor (1). The bottom leg is also bent at the knee with the side of the leg resting on the floor. Feet are placed near one another. The hand of the bottom arm is placed flat on the floor slightly wider than the shoulder, and fingers are pointing away from the torso. The top arm is resting on the top knee with the palm facing up. Inhaling, straighten the legs while pressing them together as you lift the hips up and bring the top arm up to a letter T position (2). Exhaling, rotate the torso toward the floor, hinge the weight of the torso onto the legs, and reach the top arm around the torso underneath the supporting arm (3). The legs should be strong and engaged as much as possible. Move the head to look toward the reaching hand. You must engage the shoulder girdle stabilizers, especially on the weight-bearing arm. Inhaling, return the arm and torso to the diagonally neutral position with the top arm again in the T position (2). Exhaling, return back down to the floor.

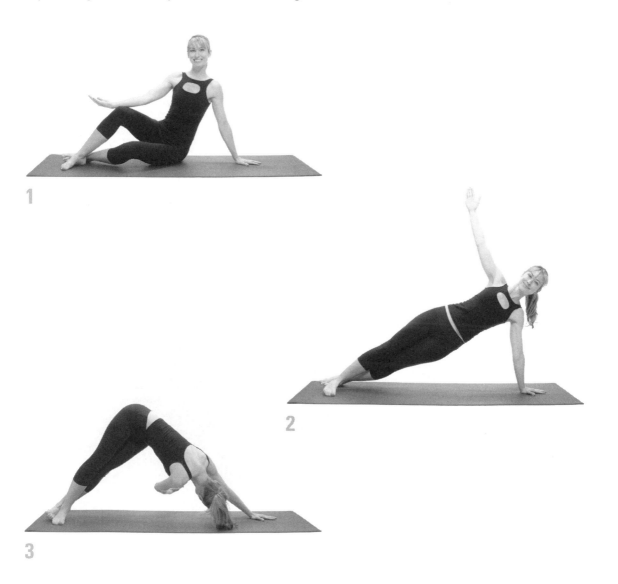

1

2

3

References

Bryant, C.X. 2005. Question and answer column. *ACE Fitness Matters Newsletter*, January/February, 14.

Douillard, J. 2001. *Body, mind, and sport: The mind-body guide to lifelong health, fitness, and your personal best.* New York: Three Rivers Press.

Ganong, W.F. 2005. *Review of medical physiology.* 22nd ed. New York: McGraw-Hill.

Howard, P.J. 2006. *The owner's manual for the brain: Everyday applications from mind–brain research.* 3rd ed. Austin: Bard Press.

McAuliffe, Kathleen. 2005. Enjoy! *U.S. News*, December 19, 2005. www.usnews.com/usnews/health/articles/051219/19coffee.htm (accessed June 2, 2006).

Pilates, J., and W.J. Miller.1998. *Pilates' return to life through contrology.* Ed. J. Robbins. Incline Village, NV: Presentation Dynamics. (Orig. pub. 1945.)

Selye, H., ed. 1980. *Selye's guide to stress research.* Vol. 1. New York: Van Nostrand Reinhold.

Spiegel, K., E. Tasali, P. Penev, and E. Van Cauter. 2004. Brief communication: Sleep curtailment in healthy young men is associated with decreased leptin levels, elevated ghrelin levels, and increased hunger and appetite. *Annals of Internal Medicine,* 141:846–850.

Taheri, S., L. Lin, D. Austin, T. Young, and E. Mignot. 2004. Short sleep duration is associated with reduced leptin, elevated ghrelin, and increased body mass index. *The Public Library of Science and Medicine* 1, no. 3 (December): e62. http://medicine.plosjournals.org/perlserv/?request=get-document&doi=10.1371/journal.pmed.0010062 (accessed June 2, 2006).

Note: The italicized *f* following a page number denotes a figure on that page.

About the Author

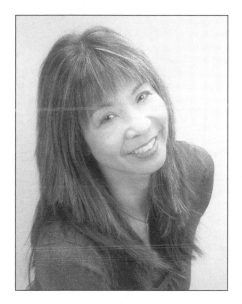

Cathleen Murakami is the owner and director of SynergySystems Fitness Studio in Encinitas, California. A professional fitness instructor for more than 20 years, she has specialized in the Pilates approach since 1991. Murakami has been a Pilates certification course instructor for more than a decade, teaching extensive anatomy, biomechanics, and rehabilitation as they relate to this method. She has also produced *The Total Fitness Workout* series of four instructional videos and DVDs that teach introductory- to intermediate-level Pilates. Murakami is **Gyrotonic** level 1 certified and also holds certifications from American Council on Exercise (ACE), American College of Sports Medicine (ACSM), Alan Herdman Pilates Studio of London, Physicalmind, and Long Beach Dance Conditioning. She has also studied yoga under Tim Miller and Erich Schiffman. Murakami resides in Encinitas, California.

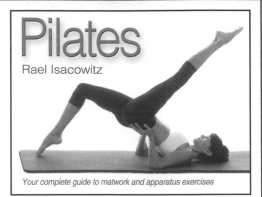
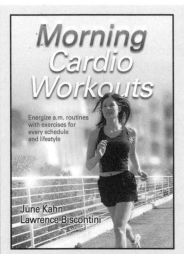
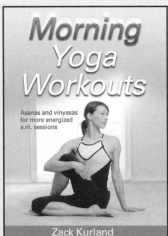
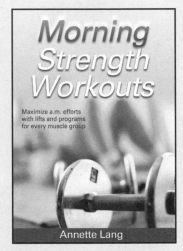